Clinical Research in Paediatric Psychopharmacology

Woodhead Publishing Series in Biomedicine

Clinical Research in Paediatric Psychopharmacology

A practical overview of the ethical, scientific, and regulatory aspects

Edited By

Philippe Auby

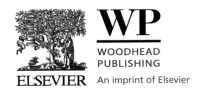

Woodhead Publishing is an imprint of Elsevier
The Officers' Mess Business Centre, Royston Road, Duxford, CB22 4QH, United Kingdom
50 Hampshire Street, 5th Floor, Cambridge, MA 02139, United States
The Boulevard, Langford Lane, Kidlington, OX5 1GB, United Kingdom

Copyright © 2020 Philippe Auby. Published by Elsevier Ltd. All rights reserved.

No part of this publication may be reproduced or transmitted in any form or by any means, electronic or mechanical, including photocopying, recording, or any information storage and retrieval system, without permission in writing from the publisher. Details on how to seek permission, further information about the Publisher's permissions policies and our arrangements with organizations such as the Copyright Clearance Center and the Copyright Licensing Agency, can be found at our website: www.elsevier.com/permissions.

This book and the individual contributions contained in it are protected under copyright by the Publisher (other than as may be noted herein).

Notices
Knowledge and best practice in this field are constantly changing. As new research and experience broaden our understanding, changes in research methods, professional practices, or medical treatment may become necessary.

Practitioners and researchers must always rely on their own experience and knowledge in evaluating and using any information, methods, compounds, or experiments described herein. In using such information or methods they should be mindful of their own safety and the safety of others, including parties for whom they have a professional responsibility.

To the fullest extent of the law, neither the Publisher nor the authors, contributors, or editors, assume any liability for any injury and/or damage to persons or property as a matter of products liability, negligence or otherwise, or from any use or operation of any methods, products, instructions, or ideas contained in the material herein.

Library of Congress Cataloging-in-Publication Data
A catalog record for this book is available from the Library of Congress

British Library Cataloguing-in-Publication Data
A catalogue record for this book is available from the British Library

ISBN: 978-0-08-100616-0 (print)
ISBN: 978-0-08-100617-7 (online)

For information on all Woodhead publications
visit our website at https://www.elsevier.com/books-and-journals

Publisher: Candice Janco
Acquisition Editor: Erin Hill-Parks
Editorial Project Manager: Michelle W. Fisher
Production Project Manager: Debasish Ghosh
Cover Designer: Mark Rogers

Typeset by SPi Global, India

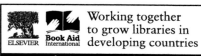

Epigraph

Science sans conscience n'est que ruine de l'âme - Science without conscience is but the ruin of the soul

Rabelais, in Pantagruel, 1532

There can be no keener revelation of a society's soul than the way in which it treats its children

Nelson Mandela, 1995

Contents

Contributors		xi
1	**Introduction** *Philippe Auby*	1
2	**Historical perspective** *Philippe Auby*	5
	2.1 Introduction	5
	2.2 Historical perspective	5
	References	12
	Further reading	13
3	**Worldwide paediatric regulations** *Philippe Auby*	15
	3.1 Introduction	15
	3.2 History of worldwide paediatric regulation	15
	3.3 Key features of US and EU paediatric regulations	21
	References	38
	Further reading	38
4	**Are the paediatric rewards adapted?** *Geneviève Michaux, Beatrice Stirner*	39
	4.1 Scope of application of the paediatric obligation	41
	4.2 Types paediatric rewards	42
	4.3 Are the paediatric rewards adapted?	58
	4.4 Switzerland	59
5	**Child and adolescent psychopharmacology at the beginning of the 21st century** *Anna I Parachikova, Philippe Auby*	67
	5.1 Introduction	67
	5.2 Historical and cultural perspective	68
	5.3 Development of child and adolescent treatments	69
	5.4 Challenges in child and adolescent psychopharmacology	70
	5.5 Unmet needs in child and adolescent pharmacology	70

	5.6 Translational disease platform	72
	5.7 Conclusion	74
	References	75
6	**Ethical aspects of research in paediatric psychopharmacology**	**81**
	Philippe Auby, Jelena Ivkovic	
	6.1 Introduction	81
	6.2 Historical perspective on ethics	81
	6.3 General ethical considerations	88
	6.4 Conclusion	97
	References	97
	Further reading	98
7	**Study design and methodology**	**99**
	Philippe Auby	
	7.1 Introduction	99
	7.2 ICE 11, the reference for paediatric research	99
	7.3 Evolving nature of study design and methodology	102
	7.4 Fundamental paediatric principles of study design and methodology	105
	7.5 Discussion: practical points to consider when designing a paediatric study	106
	7.6 Conclusion	111
	References	111
	Further reading	112
8	**Special challenges in paediatric recruitment**	**113**
	Karel Allegaert, Philippe Auby	
	8.1 Introduction	113
	8.2 Why an ethical sound paediatric recruitment strategy should be the rule?	113
	8.3 Stakeholders involved in paediatric recruitment and retention	115
	8.4 Trial design	118
	8.5 Discussion: paediatric trials on trial	118
	8.6 Conclusion	119
	References	119
	Further reading	120
	In Memoriam: Professor Dr. Klaudius Siegfried	**121**
9	**The issue of indiscriminative efficacy trials and placebo effects in paediatric psychopharmacology**	**123**
	Klaudius Siegfried	
	9.1 Introduction	123
	9.2 Basic concepts, definitions, and methodological considerations	124
	9.3 An illustration of the issue of placebo effects and false-negative indiscriminative efficacy results in paediatric psychopharmacology – Efficacy studies with antidepressants in depressive disorder	127

	9.4 Magnitude and range of placebo response in adult and paediatric populations with different mental disorders	132
	9.5 Factors of placebo effects	134
	9.6 Measures to reduce the number of indiscriminative (false-negative) efficacy studies in paediatric psychopharmacology	143
	9.7 Conclusion	146
	References	147
	Further reading	151
10	**Running clinical trials in paediatric psychopharmacology**	**153**
	Klaudius Siegfried	
	10.1 Introduction	153
	10.2 Overview of essential study management tasks and the operational plan	153
	10.3 The impact of attitudes towards paediatric psychopharmacology trials on patient availability and recruitment	156
	10.4 Challenges in the approval of studies by local regulatory authorities and IRBs/ECs	158
	10.5 Considerations on patient recruitment times and country and site selection	160
	10.6 Considerations on patient recruitment strategies	163
	10.7 Considering operational consequences of study protocol features	165
	10.8 Specific aspects of study monitoring	169
	10.9 Conclusion	171
	References	172
11	**Listening to the patients' voice**	**173**
	Deborah Lee	
	11.1 Introduction	173
	11.2 Soliciting patient/caregiver/caregiver perspective	173
	11.3 Regulatory agencies (FDA)	174
	11.4 Academic associations	176
	11.5 Pharmaceutical companies	176
	11.6 Payer groups (health technology assessments)	177
	11.7 Patients: Direct to legislation	178
	11.8 Conclusion	181
	References	181
	Further reading	182
12	**Specificities of safety management in paediatric psychopharmacological research**	**183**
	Jelena Ivkovic	
	12.1 Introduction	183
	12.2 General considerations	183
	12.3 Investigating safety and tolerability in paediatric clinical trials, points to consider	184
	12.4 ADRs in paediatric population	185

	12.5 Safety monitoring in paediatric psychopharmacological clinical trials	**186**
	12.6 Challenges and limitations of safety assessment in paediatric clinical studies	**187**
	12.7 Safety oversight, independent monitoring	**189**
	12.8 Conclusion	**189**
	References	**189**
13	**Why do we need to publish paediatric data?**	**191**
	Philippe Auby	
	13.1 Introduction	**191**
	13.2 Publishing paediatric data	**191**
	13.3 The European paediatric regulation emphasises the need to make paediatric information available to the public	**192**
	13.4 The recent rise of the antivaccine movement: Is there a link between vaccination and autism?	**194**
	13.5 Was the overall publication of paediatric MDD studies with selective serotonin reuptake inhibitors optimal?	**195**
	13.6 Conclusion	**199**
	References	**199**
	Further reading	**200**
Conclusion		**201**
Index		**203**

Contributors

Karel Allegaert Department of Pediatrics, Division of Neonatology, Erasmus MC-Sophia Children's Hospital, Rotterdam, The Netherlands; Department of Development and Regeneration, KU Leuven, Leuven, Belgium

Philippe Auby Otsuka Pharmaceutical Development & Commercialisation Europe, Frankfurt am Main, Germany

Jelena Ivkovic Senior Medical Specialist, Early Psychiatry Projects, H. Lundbeck A/S, Copenhagen, Denmark

Deborah Lee AlaWai Neurology Consulting LLC, Honolulu, HI, United States

Geneviève Michaux Mayer Brown LLP, Brussels, Belgium

Anna I Parachikova UCB Nordic A/S, Neurology Business Unit, Copenhagen, Denmark

Klaudius Siegfried Goethe Univ. Frankfurt, Frankfurt, Germany

Beatrice Stirner Swiss Federal Institute of Intellectual Property, Bern, Switzerland

Introduction

Philippe Auby
Otsuka Pharmaceutical Development & Commercialisation Europe,
Frankfurt am Main, Germany

This book is about ambition and passion.

The ambition of contributing to bringing better and innovative psychopharmacological therapies for children and adolescents as, despite significant needs for curative and preventive options in the field of child and adolescent psychiatry, presently available pharmacological treatment options are dramatically limited (Persico et al., 2015).

The passion for sharing our various professional experiences and the lessons we learned on the different programmes we participated in, to help future research and development activities.

Of course, ambition and passion are also nourished by the complexities and controversies of paediatric psychopharmacology, and this book is not aiming to give "ready to use" recipes, but this practical guide aims to share experience and best practices to support scientifically and ethically sound clinical research in paediatric psychopharmacology.

Despite significant progress over the past 20 years, paediatric psychopharmacological armamentarium remains dramatically limited, despite empirical observations and scientific data undoubtedly confirming that children and adolescents do not necessarily respond to psychopharmacological treatment like adults. If child mortality has been decreasing in almost all countries, some research shows that further to better recognition of paediatric mental disorders, mental health is worsening among the young generation. Furthermore, it appears that research in paediatric psychopharmacology remains mainly driven by commercial values, reflecting more the needs of the adults rather than those of children and adolescents due to the lower number of paediatric patients.

So, do we have sufficient ambition for our children?

To date, no pharmacological agent is aiming to treat core symptoms of autism spectrum disorder (ASD), and various medications are to reduce or control behavioural or emotional symptoms, often with limited supportive scientific data.

In 2017 the World Health Organization published a new report revealing that after road traffic injuries and lower respiratory infections, suicide and accidental death from self-harm remain the third cause of adolescent mortality in 2015 resulting in around 67,000 deaths worldwide. "Self-harm largely occurs among older adolescents, and globally, it is the second leading cause of death for older adolescent girls. It is the leading or second cause of adolescent death in Europe and South East Asia" (WHO, 2017).

Despite epidemiological studies estimating high prevalence of major depressive disorder (MDD), with the large National Comorbidity Survey-Adolescent Supplement (NCS-A) showing lifetime and 12-month prevalences of MDD up to 11.0% and 7.5%, respectively, in adolescents aged 13–18 years (Avenevoli et al., 2015), to date, only two antidepressants (two selective serotonin uptake inhibitors (SSRIs)) are approved for MDD, fluoxetine in the United States and EU in children and adolescents and escitalopram in the United States in adolescents.

This example illustrates well why child and adolescent psychiatrists are often using drugs off-label compared with adult psychiatrists who, for instance, can choose among more than 20 antidepressants and what would be the most appropriate treatment for their depressed patients.

Furthermore, we shared the vision expressed by Persico et al. that paediatric psychopharmacology holds great promise in two equally important areas of enormous biomedical and social impact, namely, the treatment of behavioural abnormalities in children and adolescents and the prevention of psychiatric disorders with adolescent or adult onset (Persico et al., 2015).

Significant unmet needs in child and adolescent psychopharmacology (from Persico et al., 2015)

The most important currently unmet needs in paediatric psychopharmacology are

- the frequent off-label prescription of medications to children and adolescents based exclusively on data from randomized controlled studies involving adult patients;
- the frequent lack of age-specific dose, long-term efficacy, and tolerability/safety data;
- the lack of effective medications for many paediatric psychiatric disorders, most critically autism spectrum disorder;
- the scarcity and limitations of randomized placebo-controlled trials in paediatric psychopharmacology;
- the unexplored potential for the prevention of psychiatric disorders with adolescent and adult onset;
- the current lack of biomarkers to predict treatment response and severe adverse effects;
- the need for better preclinical data to foster the successful development of novel drug therapies;
- the effective dissemination of evidence-based treatments to the general public, to better inform patients and families of the benefits and risks of pharmacological interventions during development.

Given the nature of the unmet needs well summarised earlier, we can confidently "claim" that paediatric clinical studies will still be necessary for the field psychopharmacology, certainly less of them, certainly different than what we have witnessed over the past years as extrapolation, modelling, and simulation will influence our clinical trial design and practices.

Is it realistic to believe that at a certain point, we will be able to avoid exposing paediatric patients to clinical trials? Probably not or not for a while.

However, aiming to reduce the number of efficacy trials seems quite achievable, while real-world evidence (RWE) studies may provide the necessary tolerability and safety information.

We further believe that the digital revolution that starts to happen in medicine offers a significant opportunity for paediatric mental health and will also transform and enhance the way children and adolescents will be treated and monitored, opening new venues for pharmacological and psychotherapeutic strategies and generating new and innovative research.

Precision medicine which has transformed some medical specialities, like oncology, may also hold significant promises for child and adolescent psychiatry despite complex challenges.

Paediatric development dramatically changed over the last years, pushing the ICH to publish in 2017 and addendum to its 2000 first guideline and will continue to change, oscillating between the necessary and sometimes mandatory studies and the critical ethical requirement to limit burden for children.

Clinical studies will continue to be necessary and conducted, mandating intransigent ethics and science.

Last but not least, we also firmly believe that one of the key challenges of future research and development is to successfully conduct a user involvement revolution, that is, like Trivedi and Wykes (2002) moving away from passive research subjects to equal partners, therefore the "Listening to the Patients' Voice" chapter where Chance, a person with autism, is sharing his story both as a 7-year-old child and later as an adult.

References

Avenevoli, S., Swendsen, J., He, J.P., Burstein, M., Merikangas, K.R., 2015. Major depression in the national comorbidity survey-adolescent supplement: prevalence, correlates, and treatment. J. Am. Acad. Child Adolesc. Psychiatry 54, 37–44. e32.

Persico, A.M., Arango, C., Buitelaar, J.K., Correll, C.U., Glennon, J.C., Hoekstra, P.J., Moreno, C., Vitiello, B., Vorstman, J., Zuddas, A., the European Child and Adolescent Clinical Psychopharmacology Network, 2015. Unmet needs in paediatric psychopharmacology: present scenario and future perspectives. Eur. Neuropsychopharmacol. 25 (10), 1513–1531.

Trivedi, P., Wykes, T., 2002. From passive subjects to equal partners: qualitative review of user involvement in research. Br. J. Psychiatry 181 (6), 468–472.

World Health Organization, 2017. http://www.who.int/mediacentre/news/releases/2017/yearly-adolescent-deaths/en/.

Historical perspective

2

Philippe Auby
Otsuka Pharmaceutical Development & Commercialisation Europe,
Frankfurt am Main, Germany

2.1 Introduction

Mental disorders in children and adolescents lead to a significant burden for them and their families, and pharmacological treatments have been slowly introduced essentially based on adult experiences and subsequent questionable or nonstrongly scientifically driven extrapolations.

Since the 1990s, first with the introduction of the selective serotonin reuptake inhibitors (SSRIs) and then with the second-generation antipsychotics (SGA), constant increased use of psychotropic agents in the paediatric population has been witnessed. Such generalised off-label prescriptions lead to legitimate worries because of the lack of robust scientific data.

Considering that, nowadays, it is unethical to deny children and adolescents access to new or innovative medications, the need to obtain paediatric information for medicines used in children seems a matter of consensus on a global basis.

Paediatric regulations, both in the US and in the EU, have played a significant role in transforming drug development, since the end of the 20th century, helping the concern of protecting children against clinical research that is fading away and promoting new paradigms, that is, protecting children through clinical research and embracing new models of drug development.

2.2 Historical perspective

2.2.1 Paediatric psychopharmacology

David Macht introduced the word 'psychopharmacology' in 1920 by, in the title of his article, describing the effects of the antipyretics, quinine and acetylsalicylic acid, on neuromuscular coordination tests.

In the 1950s, chlorpromazine was discovered and first used in the psychiatric wards in Paris. The revolutionary discovery of chlorpromazine is considered as the breakthrough in psychopharmacology, which drove the development of neuropsychopharmacology, and Henri Laborit, Pierre Deniker, and Heinz Lehmann have been awarded the Albert Lasker Award by the American Public Health Association in 1957. However, the inception of modern psychopharmacology would not have been possible without the research conducted by Charles Bradley. His observation in 1937 that children with behaviour problems showed a 'spectacular change in behaviour and remarkably improved school performance' during 1 week of treatment with benzedrine (Bradley, 1937) established the benefit of psychostimulants in the treatment of attention deficit hyperactivity disorder (ADHD). Interestingly, Bradley's work leads that the treatment of ADHD predated the use of antibiotics and his discovery profoundly influenced the field as stimulants are still the most widely prescribed psychopharmacological treatment in children (Pliska, 2012).

However, despite this early 'paediatric' breakthrough, the gap between the overall scientific knowledge and the amount of available clinical studies data between adult and paediatric psychopharmacology remains significant, with paediatric research following adult development.

It is not a surprise if ADHD is the childhood disorder for which the therapeutic armamentarium seems the more substantial, still dominated by the psychostimulants (methylphenidate and amphetamines) with limited space taken by nonstimulants (mainly atomoxetine, guanfacine, and clonidine). Research has to date failed to bring a nonstimulant that would be as effective as stimulants on core ADHD symptoms and that would also address some of the comorbid conditions or symptoms. In ADHD contrary to other fields, it is in adults rather than in children that the off-label use could be seen as a concern due to the late recognition of this disorder in adults, or more precisely the lack of awareness that ADHD was not simply vanishing in adulthood.

As reported in other chapters, there are very few psychotropic agents approved in the United States and the European Union for paediatric conditions, and the consensus is that they are not only too few in numbers but also in their targets with disorders for which there is no validated pharmacological approach.

The few approved antidepressants both in the United States or the European Union illustrate the current limitations of paediatric research and development, as understanding about their questionable efficacy, especially in depression, remains limited, while the suicidality concern originated from paediatric data has been a growing topic:

Let us first consider major depressive disorder (MDD).

Obviously, the literature about pharmacological treatment targeting paediatric MDD has grown significantly, mainly driven by the hopes raised by the introduction of the SSRIs and the development of the availability of efficacious cognitive behaviour therapy (CBT); however, it is widely acknowledged that the current evidence base is manifestly inadequate to the task of guiding best practice treatment in paediatric psychiatry.

Despite official recognition of depression in children and adolescents in Europe in 1971, when the Union of European Child and Adolescent Psychiatrists declared that depression is a critical illness, up to date, only one antidepressant is approved in the European Union, that is, fluoxetine.

Fluoxetine, also approved by the US Food and Drug Administration (FDA), is the only antidepressant available worldwide for patients >8 years of age.

In the United States, one additional SSRI, escitalopram, is approved for adolescents only, over 12 years of age.

The situation is not much better for anxiety disorders.

For generalised anxiety disorder (GAD), duloxetine is the sole drug approved for patients >7 years of age and in the United States only (note that duloxetine trials failed to separate the therapeutic agent from placebo in the depression programme).

For obsessive-compulsive disorders (OCD), fluvoxamine and sertraline were approved globally for quite some years with initial paediatric written requests issued by the FDA in 1999, and unfortunately despite therapeutic needs, since then, no significant pharmacological research has been performed in paediatric OCD.

Schizophrenia and paediatric bipolar I disorder have been subject to more therapeutic investigations over the recent years.

Actually, since the introduction of the often called second-generation antipsychotics, more extensive paediatric research in the paediatric population has been reported, triggered mainly by the FDA with the issue of paediatric written requests and more recently by the EU paediatric regulation. Research occurred essentially in adolescents with schizophrenia and to a lesser extent in younger patients with paediatric bipolar disorder, that is, mania.

Significantly less research occurred in behavioural disorders.

Currently, oral formulations of several atypical antipsychotics (risperidone, olanzapine, quetiapine, aripiprazole, and paliperidone) are approved for use in children and adolescents for treatment of schizophrenia and bipolar I disorder fostering the overall increased use of these agents in the paediatric population. In the United States, the use of antipsychotics in adolescents and young adults (14–20 years old) has shown a nearly fivefold increase between the periods 1993–98 and 2005–09 (Olfson et al., 2010).

Interestingly, safety data revealed that paediatric patients, especially naive ones, are at higher risk than adults for experiencing adverse events.

Consequently, in 2013, the American Psychiatric Association decided to warn about their paediatric use outside the approved indications (Table 2.1).

To date, in Europe, very few psychotropic medications have been approved for use in children and adolescents, as illustrated in Table 2.2 adapted from Persico et al. (2015) and updated with the additional approvals that occurred until end of 2018.

Actually the majority of medications used worldwide to treat child and adolescent psychiatric conditions remain probably unlicensed and off-label.

These paediatric gaps between needs and research, use, and data raise an inevitable question:

2.2.2 Why so limited research?

Several reasons have been reported in the literature to explain the lack of research; among them, we can cite the following:

1) Research has not always been promoted and even have been discouraged, for instance, by a certain vision of psychoanalysis, which used to dominate the field of child and adolescent psychiatry.
(2) There have been some persisting taboos about paediatric psychopharmacology. For instance, the concern of overmedicating children should have stimulated strong scientific projects to bring valuable information but was instead used to discourage paediatric research.

Table 2.1 APA 2013

Do not routinely prescribe an antipsychotic medication to treat behavioural and emotional symptoms of childhood mental disorders in the absence of approved or evidence-supported indications
There are both on- and off-label clinical indications for antipsychotic drug use in children and adolescents. The FDA-approved and/or evidence-supported indications for antipsychotic medications in children and adolescents include psychotic disorders, bipolar disorder, tic disorders, and severe irritability in children with autism spectrum disorders; there is increasing evidence that antipsychotic medications may be useful for some disruptive behaviour disorders. Children and adolescents should be prescribed antipsychotic medications only after having had a careful diagnostic assessment with attention to comorbid medical conditions and a review of the patient's prior treatments. Efforts should be made to combine both evidence-based pharmacological and psychosocial interventions and support. Limited availability of evidence-based psychosocial interventions may make it difficult for every child to receive this ideal combination. Discussion of potential risks and benefits of medication treatment with the child and their guardian is critical. A short- and long-term treatment and monitoring plan to assess outcome, side effects, metabolic status, and discontinuation, if appropriate, is also critical. The evidence base for use of atypical antipsychotics in preschool and younger children is limited, and therefore further caution is warranted in prescribing in this population
http://www.choosingwisely.org/societies/american-psychiatric-association

(3) Paediatric research is often perceived as too complicated. Despite being often more complex and more difficult than research in adults, as illustrated by the more complicated consent/assent process, it is however achievable and highly valuable.
(4) Paediatric population may be small, for instance, schizophrenia below the age of 15 years of age or major depressive disorder in children, making it challenging to conduct large efficacy studies.
(5) Without neglecting true ethical barriers, these concerns have sometimes been instrumentalised as a basis not to conduct research, promoting the need to protect children from research, despite the evidence pointing out that paediatric clinical trials could be instrumental in modifying the outcome of paediatric disorders by bringing new and innovative therapeutic options. Childhood vaccine development is undoubtedly the most striking example of primary paediatric prevention.
(6) Finally, research is expensive, and paediatric research even more. The lack of commercial incentive being more the rule than the exception has been well recognised in the United States and Europe, leading to the incorporation of financial incentives or rewards in both regulations. The costs associated with the development of specific age-adjusted paediatric formulation are often used as an illustration of the additional burden of paediatric development.

2.2.3 Are paediatric studies still necessary?

The answer seems simple. Yes, studies are still necessary as discussed previously in this chapter, but their real necessity must always thoroughly be assessed.

Table 2.2 Psychotropic medications approved in Europe for use in children and adolescents

Medication	Indication	Age for prescription (years)
Aripiprazole	Schizophrenia	≥15
	Bipolar disorder, manic or mixed episodes	≥13
Amphetamines (including Lisdexamfetamine)	Attention deficit hyperactivity disorder[a]	≥6
Atomoxetine	Attention deficit hyperactivity disorder	≥6
Fluoxetine	Major depressive episode	≥8
Fluvoxamine	Obsessive-compulsive disorder	≥8
Methylphenidate	Attention deficit hyperactivity disorder	≥6
Risperidone	Aggression[b]	≥5
Sertraline	Obsessive-compulsive disorder	≥6
Ziprasidone	Bipolar disorder, manic or mixed episode[c]	≥10
Paliperidone	Schizophrenia	≥15
Melatonin	Insomnia is ASD	≥2
Guanfacine	Attention deficit hyperactivity disorder	≥6

Adapted from Persico, A.M., Arango, C., Buitelaar, J.K., Correll, Ch.U., Glennon, J.C., Hoekstra, P.J., Moreno, C., Vitiello, B., Vorstman, J., Zuddas, A., The European Child and Adolescent Clinical Psychopharmacology Network, 2015. Unmet needs in paediatric psychopharmacology: present scenario and future perspectives. Eur. Neuropsychopharmacol. 25 (10), 1513–1531.
[a]Approved only in some European countries for children and adolescents with ADHD.
[b]Approved only in some European countries for children and adolescents with conduct disorder, in the presence of sub-average intellectual functioning or intellectual disability and when all nonpharmacological strategies have been found insufficient.
[c]Approved only in some European countries based on one randomised controlled trial (Findling et al., 2013), found by the US Food and Drug Administration to have quality assurance issues, requiring the sponsor to repeat the trial.

So, the question has always to be evaluated on a case-by-case basis: Is 'this' particular foreseen paediatric study necessary?

All clinical trials enrolling paediatric patients should be scientifically and ethically sound, aiming to answer a clinical or therapeutic question with the objective to provide robust information.

For FDA- or EMA-mandated and FDA- or EMA-regulated trials, paediatric regulations provide some guidance.

Unnecessary trials are not acceptable, and the 2006 EU paediatric regulation phrased it clearly:

These objectives (i.e. of the EU regulation) should be achieved without subjecting the paediatric population to unnecessary clinical trials and without delaying the authorisation of medicinal products for other age populations.

Extrapolations, modelling, and simulations are more and more considered.

According to ICH E11 (R1) Addendum, 'Pediatric extrapolation is defined as an approach to providing evidence in support of effective and safe use of drugs in the pediatric population when it can be assumed that the course of the disease and the expected response to a medicinal product would be sufficiently similar in the pediatric and reference (adult or other pediatric) population'. Paediatric extrapolation will be addressed in a future ICH guideline as endorsed by the ICH Assembly actually in line with the updated version of EMA's draft reflection paper on the use of extrapolation in the development of medicines for paediatrics published on October 13, 2017.

The extrapolation of efficacy from adult and other sources of information to the paediatric population minimises the risk of exposing patients to clinical trials and, by increasing the speed of drug development, may allow faster access to new medicines for paediatric. The FDA Pediatric Study Decision Tree (Fig. 2.1) is an assumption-based algorithm that provides a helpful starting point in determining the need and, if deemed necessary, the nature of required paediatric studies in paediatric drug development programmes.

For paediatric development programmes, if the assumptions needed for extrapolation do not apply (option A), then extrapolation cannot be used, and therefore efficacy has to be demonstrated and replicated in the paediatric population, usually meaning two adequate studies.

Partial extrapolation (option B) eliminates the need to conduct two efficacy trials, and one should suffice.

Complete extrapolation of efficacy from adult or other paediatric data to the paediatric population eliminates the need for paediatric efficacy trials (option C).

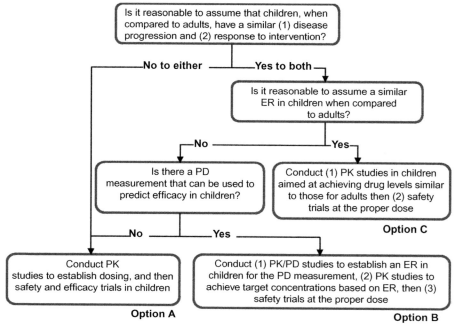

Fig. 2.1 FDA pediatric study decision tree. *ER*, exposure response.

Further to giving guidance to the industry for paediatric development programmes, this decision tree frames the critical drivers of any paediatric study, that is, 'Is there a clinical/therapeutic question that will be addressed by the planned study?'. This will be further discussed in the chapter focusing on ethical considerations pertaining to paediatric psychopharmacology research.

2.2.4 Modelling and simulation

Depending on the regions and scientific background, several names are used further to modelling and simulation (M&S) essentially model-informed drug development (MIDD) or model-informed drug discovery and development (MID3).

The ICH E11 addendum published in 2017 defines M&S as follows: 'Advancement in clinical pharmacology and quantitative M&S techniques has enabled progress in using model-informed approaches (e.g., mathematical/statistical models and simulations based on physiology, pathology, and pharmacology) in drug development. M&S can help quantify available information and assist in defining the design of pediatric clinical studies and/or the dosing strategy. Considering the limited ability to collect data in the pediatric population, pediatric drug development requires tools to address knowledge gaps. M&S is one such tool that can help avoid unnecessary pediatric studies and help ensure appropriate data are generated from the smallest number of pediatric patients'.

There are numerous applications for M&S as summarised by S. Rohou in Fig. 2.2; however, the current use of M&S in regulatory submission is currently limited due to lack of wide acceptance within pharmaceutical companies and uncertainties about regulator's responses (Rohou, 2017). In 2016 the EFPIA MID3 Workgroup published a white paper aiming to enable greater consistency in the practice, application,

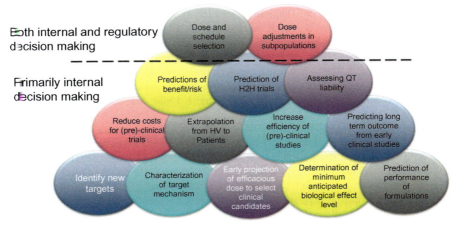

Fig. 2.2 Application of MID3 (Solange Corriol-Rohou, 2017). FDA Workshop: Pediatric Trial Design and Modeling – Moving into the next decade.

and documentation of model-informed drug discovery and development across the pharmaceutical industry with the following three major objectives (EFPIA MID3 Workgroup et al., 2016):

(1) Informing company decision-makers how the strategic integration of MID3 can benefit R&D efficiency
(2) Providing MID3 analysts with sufficient material to enhance the planning, rigour, and consistency of the application of MID3
(3) Providing regulatory authorities with substrate to develop MID3-related and/or MID3-enabled guidelines.

2.2.5 Conclusion

2.2.5.1 Will we continue performing paediatric studies?

Probably!

Dose-finding and safety studies in paediatric patients will probably still be needed for some years.

However, some efficacy studies that have been considered as necessary until now will certainly no longer be necessary.

2.2.5.2 Take the opportunity to contribute!

This is your white page, feel free to write on it....

References

Bradley, C., 1937. The behavior of children receiving benzedrine. Am. J. Psychiatry 94, 577–585.
EFPIA MID3 Workgroup, Marshall, S.F., Burghaus, R., Cosson, V., Cheung, S.Y.A., Chenel, M., DellaPasqua, O., Frey, N., Hamren, B., Harnisch, L., Ivanow, F., Kerbusch, T., Lippert, J., Milligan, P.A., Rohou, S., Staab, A., Steimer, J.L., Tornøe, C., Visser, S.A.G., 2016. Good practices in model-informed drug discovery and development: practice, application, and documentation. CPT Pharmacometrics Syst. Pharmacol. 5, 93–122.
Findling, R.L., Cavuş, I., Pappadopulos, E., Vanderburg, D.G., Schwartz, J.H., Gundapaneni. B.K., DelBello, M.P., 2013. Efficacy, long-term safety, and tolerability of ziprasidone in children and adolescents with bipolar disorder. J. Child. Adolesc. Psychopharmacol. 23 (8), 531–544.
Olfson, M., Crystal, S., Huang, C., Gerhard, T., 2010. Trends in antipsychotic drug use by very young, privately insured children. J. Am. Acad. Child Adolesc. Psychiatry 49, 13–23.
Persico, A.M., Arango, C., Buitelaar, J.K., Correll, C.U., Glennon, J.C., Hoekstra, P.J., Moreno, C., Vitiello, B., Vorstman, J., Zuddas, A., The European Child and Adolescent Clinical Psychopharmacology Network, 2015. Unmet needs in paediatric psychopharmacology: present scenario and future perspectives. Eur. Neuropsychopharmacol. 25 (10), 1513–1531.
Pliska, S.R., 2012. In: Rosenberg, D.R., Gershon, S. (Eds.), Psychostimulants in Pharmacotherapy of Child and Adolescent Psychiatric Disorders, third ed. Wiley-Blackwell.

Rohou, S., 2017. ICH E11 revisions and pediatric model informed drug development and simulation. In: FDA 2017 workshop Pediatric Trial Design and Modeling: Moving Into the Next Decade. https://www.fda.gov/Drugs/NewsEvents/ucm564111.htm.

Further reading

Ban, A.T., 2007. Fifty years chlorpromazine: a historical perspective. Neuropsychiatr. Dis. Treat. 3 (4), 495–500.

ICH E11 addendum, https://www.fda.gov/downloads/Drugs/GuidanceComplianceRegulatoryInformation/Guidances/UCM530012.pdf.

Worldwide paediatric regulations

Philippe Auby
Otsuka Pharmaceutical Development & Commercialisation Europe,
Frankfurt am Main, Germany

3.1 Introduction

It seems nowadays beyond any reasonable doubt that the need to obtain specific information for medicines used in the paediatric population and the urge to develop innovative drugs for patients below 18 years of age have reached a consensus on a global basis (Auby, 2014). This statement would not have been possible without the existence of two major paediatric regulations, the first one in the United States and the second in EU, and the work of the International Council for Harmonisation of Technical Requirements for Pharmaceuticals for Human Use with the ICH E11.

If the United States paved the way for legislation aimed at producing drugs for children, followed more recently by the EU, further initiatives or paediatric considerations are taking place globally as evidenced by the recent Swiss initiative described in more details in the following chapter of this book or by the circular that the Chinese Government released in 2014 on ensuring drug safety for children, raising requirements in various aspects such as research and development, supply, and quality management.

We also strongly believe that parents should be precisely informed if a medicinal product will be prescribed off-label to their child when making a decision.

The 'paediatric regulations' will be covered by two distinct chapters starting with this first chapter, the voluntary 'descriptive' part, focusing on the key features of these regulations, with the objective to provide sufficient insight to understand both regulations, followed by a second chapter, the 'analytic' one, providing a deep dive in the intricacies of the paediatric rewards for both the EU and the Swiss paediatric regulations.

3.2 History of worldwide paediatric regulation

3.2.1 US paediatric regulation

Paediatric clinical drug testing legislation originates almost 200 years ago; from the 19th century, with the creation of the AMA Women and Children' Division and the American Academy of Paediatrics, Rivera and Hartzema remind us that 'paediatric drug development was always guided by public policy and had a long history of successes and failures' (Rivera). As an example, they consider the National Childhood Vaccine Injury Act of 1986 as one of the reasons enabling vaccine development to continue, by creating in 1988 the National Vaccine Injury Compensation Program (VICP); this VICP was established to ensure an adequate supply of vaccines, stabilise vaccine costs, and establish and maintain an accessible and efficient forum for individuals found to be injured by certain vaccines (VICP).

The key milestone occurred in 1994 when the United States implemented the 'Paediatric Labeling Rule' that truly paved the way for legislation aimed at producing drugs for children. Since 1979, there was a paediatric use section for drugs in the United States. What this new FDA regulation brought was requiring manufacturers of marketed drugs to survey existing data and to determine whether the data were sufficient to support additional paediatric use information in the drug's labelling. If the data existed, manufacturers were encouraged to submit a supplemental NDA seeking a labelling change. If the information was insufficient, the rule required the labelling of the drug to state that 'safety and effectiveness in paediatric patients have not been established'. Since then, the legislation went through several reauthorisations and amendments.

This initiative was followed in 1997 by the FDA Modernisation Act that 'provided an incentive for pharmaceutical companies to study products for which there would be a health benefit in the paediatric population'. This created a 'voluntary process where FDA would define the products that needed paediatric studies, outline the necessary studies, and issue sponsors a Paediatric Written Request'. Pharmaceutical companies could choose to respond or not to the Paediatric Written Request, and if responding positively six additional months of marketing exclusivity were received upon completion of the agreed program. This process is considered as the key main legislative initiative that has changed paediatric drug development in the United States.

In January 2002, the Best Pharmaceuticals for Children Act (BPCA) came into force and confirmed this voluntary framework for companies to undertake studies of on-patent and off-patent drugs for use in paediatric populations in exchange for extended product exclusivity.

In 2003, the Paediatric Research Equity Act (PREA) came into force. PREA empowered the FDA to require paediatric investigation of a product for which a New Drug Application (NDA) was submitted if the agency determined that the product was likely to be used in a substantial number of paediatric patients, or if it would provide meaningful benefits for children over existing treatments.

In July 2012, the FDA Safety and Innovation Act (FDASIA) expanded the FDA's authority and strengthened the agency's ability to safeguard and advance public health by renewing the preexisting paediatric regulations and reinforcing essential laws for drugs, biologics, and medical devices including the BPCA, PREA, and Paediatric Medical Device Safety and Innovation Act. One significant additional change was the end of what was called the sunset of US paediatric regulations by making both BPCA and PREA permanent like the EU regulation that had come into force 5 years earlier and no longer subject to reauthorisation every 5 years.

3.2.2 2006 EU paediatric regulation

In Europe, a similar thought process started in the late 1990s, and in December 2000, the European Health Council asked the EU commission to take action to remedy the fact that the majority of drugs used in paediatric patients have never been tested for this specific population; this concern had been raised by regulators, individual member states, members of the European Parliament, paediatricians, and importantly also by parents representatives. The consultation paper released in 2002 called 'Better Medicines for Children' presented the European Commission reflections and positions for ambitious regulatory actions on paediatric medicines, which were used to build the future EU paediatric regulation in order to bring faster and more profound changes in EU compared with the United States. It is in this consultation paper that was emphasised that despite representing 20% of the total population in the EU, paediatric populations could be considered 'therapeutic orphans' as the majority of medicines were still only developed and assessed for adults with an estimation that at that time, up to 90% of medicinal products, depending on therapeutic areas, used in younger patients have never been specifically evaluated for such use. The 'therapeutic orphans' designation introduced by Harry Shirkey in 1962 has been quite criticised as these kids have responsible 'parents'; however his strong wording does question our collective responsibilities vis-à-vis our children to ensure they can get the best possible care: 'If we are to have drugs of better efficacy and safety for children, those responsible for child care will have to assume this responsibility for developing active programs of clinical pharmacology and drug testing in infants and children. The alternative is to accept the status of "Therapeutic Orphans" for their patients'. (Shirkey, 1999).

The first 2016 European Paediatric Regulation came into force in EU on the 26 January 2007 as before this time there was no overall regulatory framework for the development of medicines for children. Like the US paediatric regulation, its core objective is to improve the health of children in Europe by facilitating the development and availability of medicines for children aged 0–17 years, ensuring that medicines for use in children are of high quality, ethically researched, and authorised appropriately. The need for adapted paediatric formulations for the different ICH E11 age groups is emphasised in the regulation despite being often considered of a lower priority compared with the need of generating safety and efficacy data. Additionally, this regulation aims to facilitate the availability of information on the use of medicines for children, and the importance of publishing paediatric studies is developed in another chapter of the book ('Why do we need to publish paediatric data?').

Therefore, paediatric development became mandatory in EU for all new medicinal products in development unless a waiver is granted, and pharmaceutical companies have to send a paediatric investigation plan (PIP) as early as the end of pharmacokinetic studies in adults.

This new regulation aims to

- increase the development of medicines for use in children,
- ensure that medicines used to treat children are as follows:
  - subject to high-quality research
  - appropriately authorised for use in children
- improve the information available on the use of medicines in children,
- achieve the above objectives without subjecting children to unnecessary clinical trials or delaying the authorisation of medicines in the adult population.

The regulation and further background information are found at the *European Commission website*.

Fig. 3.1 summarises below the history of US and EU Paediatric Regulations.

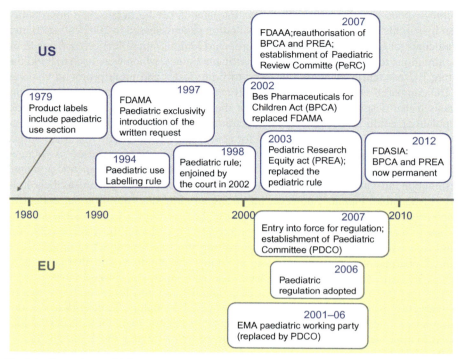

Fig 3.1 Chronology of US and EU paediatric regulations.

3.2.3 2000 ICH E11

The ICH E11 'Clinical Investigation of Medicinal Products in the Paediatric Population' came into operation in 2001 (Table 3.1). The guideline provides an outline of critical issues in paediatric drug development and approaches to the safe, efficient, and ethical study of medicinal products in the paediatric population, stating the general principles: 'Paediatric patients should be given medicines that have been appropriately evaluated for their use. Safe and effective pharmacotherapy in paediatric patients requires the timely development of information on the proper

Table 3.1 ICH E11: key dates

First codification	History	Date
E11	Approval by the Steering Committee under *Step 2* and release for public consultation	7 October 1999
E11	Approval by the Steering Committee under *Step 4* and recommendation for adoption to the three ICH regulatory bodies	19 July 2000

use of medicinal products in paediatric patients of various ages and, often, the development of paediatric formulations of those products. Advances in formulation chemistry and in paediatric study design will help facilitate the development of medicinal products for paediatric use. Drug development programs should usually include the paediatric patient population when a product is being developed for a disease or condition in adults and it is anticipated the product will be used in the paediatric population. Obtaining knowledge of the effects of medicinal products in paediatric patients is an important goal. However, this should be done without compromising the well-being of paediatric patients participating in clinical studies. This responsibility is shared by companies, regulatory authorities, health professionals, and society as a whole'.

Fifteen years later, in 2017, the ICH published an addendum (R1) to ICH E11: 'Paediatric drug development has evolved since the original ICH E11 Guideline (2000), requiring consideration of regulatory and scientific advances relevant to paediatric populations. This addendum does not alter the scope of the original guideline which outlines an approach to the safe, efficient, and ethical study of medicinal products in the paediatric population. ICH E11 (2000), including the present addendum (R1) is not intended to be comprehensive; other ICH guidelines, as well as documents from regulatory authorities worldwide, the World Health Organization (WHO) and paediatric societies, provide additional detail. The purpose of this addendum is to complement and provide clarification and current regulatory perspective on topics in paediatric drug development...'

In particular, E11 (R1) addendum supplements the current E11 guideline in extrapolation, modelling and simulation, and trial methodology.

While ICH emphasised that a full revision of the guideline is not currently deemed necessary, the principles of the ICH E11 remains clear (Table 3.2).

The ICH E11 provides a common classification of the paediatric population into age categories (Table 3.3). Of course, any classification is to some extent arbitrary, but it offers a basis for thinking about study design in paediatric patients. Depending on factors such as the condition, the treatment, and the study design, it may be justifiable to include paediatric subpopulations in adult studies or adult subpopulations in paediatric studies.

Table 3.2 ICHE11 principles

Principles of ICH E11
• Paediatric patients should be given medicines that have been properly evaluated for their use in the intended population
• Product development programmes should include paediatric studies when paediatric use is anticipated
• Development of product information in paediatric patients should be timely and often requires the development of paediatric formulations
• The rights of paediatric participants should be protected, and they should be shielded from undue risk

Table 3.3 Age groups according to ICHE11

Five different paediatric age groups according to ICH E11
Preterm newborn infants
Term newborn infants (0–27 days)
Infants and toddlers (from 28 days to 23 months)
Children (2–11 years)
Adolescents (from 12 to 16–18 years)

3.2.4 WHO 'make medicines child size' campaign – 2007

In 2007, the World Health Assembly passed a resolution WHA60.20 calling for specific actions from the World Health Organization (WHO) and the member states to improve access to better medicines for children. Later that year, WHO published the first WHO Model List of Essential Medicines for Children and launched in December 2007 a campaign called 'make medicines child size'. It clearly identified the numerous challenges associated with paediatric drug development and the need for a broad involvement of pharmaceutical companies, regulatory authorities, health professionals, and society as a whole in response to these challenges (www.who.int/childmedicines/en).

Additionally, the WHO campaign emphasises the fact that this issue is a global issue, with different urgent needs depending on the countries, even in the wealthiest countries and certainly in the developing world. The issue of appropriate paediatric formulations clearly illustrates the different challenges like the pills that nurses are still crushing in fancy university hospitals to the inadequate formulation stability when facing transport logistics issues and high temperatures in other areas.

Please find below (Table 3.4) the WHO press release.

Table 3.4 "Make Medicines Child Size" December 2007 press release

6 DECEMBER 2007|LONDON/GENEVA – Efforts to ensure children have better access to medicines appropriate for them intensified today with the unveiling of a new research and development agenda by WHO. The agenda, presented at the London launch of a campaign named "Make medicines child size", targets a range of medicines – including antibiotics, asthma and pain medication – that need to be better tailored to children's needs. It calls for further research and development of combination pills for HIV/AIDS, TB and malaria, as well as appropriate child therapy for a number of neglected tropical diseases.
"The gap between the availability and the need for child-appropriate medicines touches wealthy as well as poor countries," said Dr Margaret Chan, WHO Director-General. "As we strive for equitable access to scientific progress in health, children must be one of our top priorities."
WHO has already begun work to promote increased attention to research into children's medicines. The agency is building an Internet portal to clinical trials carried out in children and will publish the web site containing that information early next year.
First list of essential medicines for children

Table 3.4 Continued

WHO is also releasing today the first international List of Essential Medicines for Children. The list contains 206 medicines that are deemed safe for children and address priority conditions. "But a lot remains to be done. There are priority medicines that have not been adapted for children's use or are not available when needed," said Dr Hans Hogerzeil, Director of Medicines Policy and Standards at WHO. In industrialized societies more than half of the children are prescribed medicines dosed for adults and not authorized for use in children. In developing countries, the problem is compounded by lower access to medicines.
Each year about 10 million children do not reach their fifth birthday. Approximately six million of these children die of treatable conditions and could be saved if the medicines they need were readily available, safe, effective and affordable.
Pneumonia alone causes approximately two million deaths in children under five each year and HIV kills 330 000 children under 15. "These illnesses can be treated but many children don't stand a chance because the medicines are either not appropriate for their age, don't reach them or are priced too high – up to three times the price of adult drugs," said Dr Howard Zucker, WHO Assistant Director-General.
WHO will also work with governments to promote changes in their legal and regulation requirements for children's medicines

3.2.5 Swiss paediatric regulatory framework – 2019

The Swiss paediatric regulatory framework will be presented and discussed in the next chapter about paediatric incentives. Ten years after the EU paediatric regulation was released, in 2016, Switzerland adopted its incentive system for paediatric medicinal products. Based on the same principle about ensuring access for children to medicines adequately tailored to their needs, the Swiss legislator introduced several measures to encourage innovation that leads to new paediatric treatments, rather than off-label uses of adult medicines. The Swiss system is implemented on the basis of EU Regulation (EC) No. 1901/2006 and introduces the obligation to develop and submit a PIP and to carry out studies for paediatric. Applicants have two options: they can either submit a PIP that has already been approved by a foreign medicines agency (for instance the European Medicines Agency or the Food and Drug Agency), with comparable medicinal product control, or they can develop their own PIP. This new and revised regulatory frame entered into force on the 1st of January 2019. It is of course too early to assess the impact of Swiss incentive system for paediatric medicinal products due to its novelty. However, by introducing new approaches, it constitutes an elegant and innovative approach that should serve as a model for other countries as additional paediatric regulations should instead add new incentives and opportunities than burden if we want to make paediatric development successful.

3.3 Key features of US and EU paediatric regulations

ICH E11, WHO, and worldwide paediatric regulations express similar regulatory expectations for paediatric drug development:

- Safety and efficacy of the drug should be studied in all appropriate age groups.
- Paediatric formulations should be developed.

- Labels should reflect the paediatric data.
- Paediatric development plans (or waivers) must be submitted early in the drug development process.

However, these expectations translate in different requirements, legal provisions, and implementation procedures.

3.3.1 Key features of the US paediatric regulatory framework

The Food and Drug Administration Safety and Innovation Act (FDASIA), signed into law on July 9, 2012, expands the FDA's authorities and strengthens the agency's ability to improve the safety and effectiveness of paediatric drugs, biological products, and medical devices used in children: the Best Pharmaceuticals for Children Act (BPCA), the Paediatric Research Equity Act (PREA), and the Paediatric Medical Device Safety and Improvement Act: 'Children have unique needs for medical products and these provisions increase the FDA's ability to meet these needs. By making BPCA and PREA permanent – no longer subject to reauthorization every five years – the law ensures that children will have a permanent place on the agenda for drug research and development'.

Without speculating about the intentionality of what triggered the FDASIA, it is essential to highlight that in 2012 the US paediatric regulation moved closer to the EU position in term of earlier rather than later paediatric development plan submission, at least for drug manufacturers subject to PREA. Indeed, FDASIA amends PREA to require submission of paediatric study plans no later than 60 days after an end-of-phase 2 (EOP 2) meeting with the FDA or at a time agreed upon with FDA. The content and process for initial paediatric study plans (iPSP) and amendments to agreed iPSP are described in the FDASIA.

These new features give additional authority to the FDA to speed paediatric drug information to patients, health care professionals and society as a whole.

The US paediatric regulations, that is, both the PREA and BPCA, apply to New Drug Applications (NDAs) and Biologics License Applications (BLAs) but differ in their provisions.

3.3.1.1 Paediatric Research Equity Act (PREA)

PREA requires paediatric assessments of certain drugs and biological products only in the adult indications that are approved or for which the sponsor is seeking approval. PREA is triggered when an application or supplement is submitted for a new indication, new dosing regimen, new active ingredient, new dosage form, and/or a new route of administration.

It does not apply for orphan indications.

It also can be invoked by FDA for a product for which an application or supplement is not being submitted if a Written Request issued under BPCA has been declined by the sponsor and other BPCA-created mechanisms to obtain that the studies have been exhausted. PREA includes provisions allowing FDA to defer or waive the required paediatric assessments under limited circumstances. The FDASIA requires earlier PSP submission by drug manufacturers subject to PREA and gives FDA new authority to help ensure that PREA requirements are addressed in a timely fashion. Effective since July 2013, applicants are required to submit their initial PSP, and information to support any planned request for waiver or deferral, not later than 60 days after the end of phase 2 or at the latest before phase 3 initiation. For products for life-threatening diseases, the appropriate review division will provide its best judgment at the end-of-phase 1 meetings on whether paediatric studies will be required under PREA and whether the submission will be deferred.

The PSP is a statement of intent that outlines the paediatric studies that the applicant plans to conduct and addresses the development of an age-appropriate formulation and whether, if so, what grounds the applicant plans to request a waiver or deferral under PREA.

The FDA review ad hoc division that handles that particular drug, or biologic provides their best judgment about

- whether a paediatric assessment is required;
- whether its submission can be deferred or waived;
- if deferred, indicating the date studies should be due.

How does a deferral work under PREA?

FDA can grant a deferral when

- additional safety and effectiveness information in adults is needed before beginning studies in children;
- the product is ready for approval in adults, but the paediatric studies cannot be completed simultaneously;
- There is another valid reason for deferral.

Plans for deferred studies must be submitted to the FDA after the end of phase 2 with the PSP and be agreed upon by the Review Division and Paediatric Review Committee (PeRC). Submission of a PSP (i.e. PK/PD, safety, and/or efficacy studies) must accompany any deferral request in an NDA/BLA submission. Studies will be conducted later in the development of the product, usually postapproval as a postmarketing requirement.

What about waivers under PREA?

PREA requirements can be waived for some or all subsets of the paediatric population based on established criteria, on the FDA own initiative or at the request of an applicant. The criteria for a full or partial waiver are similar except for the formulation criterion that only applies for partial waivers. A waiver can be granted if

- necessary studies are impossible or highly impracticable (such as when a disease or condition does not ordinarily occur in children).
- there is evidence strongly suggesting that the drug or biological product would be ineffective or unsafe.
- the drug or biological product does not represent a meaningful therapeutic benefit over existing therapies for paediatric patients and is not likely to be used in a substantial number of paediatric patients.
- Additionally, a partial waiver can be granted if an applicant can demonstrate that reasonable attempts to produce a paediatric formulation for that age group have failed. If a waiver is granted on the basis that it is not possible to develop a paediatric formulation, the waiver shall cover only the paediatric groups requiring that formulation.

PREA requires explicitly that if a full or partial waiver is granted because available evidence suggests a product would be unsafe or ineffective in children, this information must be included in the US package insert for the product.

A list of diseases that have extremely limited applicability to paediatric patients in that the signs and symptoms of these diseases occur for the most part in the adult population is found in the on the FDA website. Products being developed for the treatment of these conditions in adults are likely to be granted a waiver.

PREA process and compliance

A review and agreement to an initial PSP generally will require at least 7 months, and a PSP should ideally be submitted before phase 3 initiation. An initial agreed PSP must be in place at the time the BLA/NDA is submitted.

FDASIA amends PREA to ensure the completion of paediatric studies and authorises FDA to grant an extension of assessments deferred under PREA. This provision applies to all deferred studies, including those already considered delayed. In order to alert applicants, FDA sent reminders and may grant deferral extensions (DE) during this process of interaction with the sponsors. It is crucial to enlighten the need to interact with the FDA and be transparent about the reasons for delays in paediatric programmes (Table 3.5) as failure to demonstrate any communication with FDA about problems encountered in completing the paediatric studies may be grounds for denial of a deferral extension request.

Table 3.5 Reasons for delays in paediatric programmes

Reasons cited for DE request	Examples of scenarios associated with each reason
Delays due to issues with the study drug and/or comparator drug	Delays developing an age-appropriate formulation
	Product quality and stability issues
	Comparator drug shortage
Delays involving study participants, sites, and/or management	Difficulty recruiting study participants
	High rate of site personnel turnover
	Additional time needed to address unexpected issues in study conduct
Delays due to safety and/or pharmacokinetic issues	Additional safety data required
	Must review new pharmacokinetic data before proceeding with the study
	Study proceeding with a more cautious approach due to new potential safety signals
Delays due to continuing interaction between the applicant and FDA	FDA placed study on clinical hold
	FDA requested change in the protocol
	The applicant and FDA are negotiating a different study to fulfil the PREA requirement
Additional time required to prepare the study report and/or submission	Delays collecting and compiling study data
	Additional time required to analyze study data
	Additional time required to prepare a supplemental NDA with appropriate paediatric labeling

In addition to the authority to grant DEs for PREA-required studies, FDASIA requires FDA to send a PREA noncompliance letter to sponsors who have failed to submit their paediatric assessments required under PREA by the final due date, have failed to seek or obtain a deferral or deferral extension, or have failed to request approval for a required paediatric formulation. The legislation further requires the FDA to post the PREA noncompliance letter and sponsor's response.

3.3.1.2 Best Pharmaceutical Children Act (BPCA)

BPCA for 'on-patent' products

The goal of the BPCA process is to obtain paediatric studies that will enable a sponsor to fully label the drug for paediatric use. The BPCA is first applicable to approved NDA and BLAs with remaining patent or product exclusivity and is based on a voluntary mechanism as it can be initiated in two ways:

- Either the FDA determines there is a public health need for additional paediatric studies for a particular drug and issue a Paediatric Written Request (PWR) for such studies.
- Alternatively, a sponsor initiates the process by submitting a proposed PPSR to FDA proposing studies believed appropriate. The FDA will review the PPSR and may use it as a starting point for drafting the PWR. The FDA will not issue a PWR if they determine there is not a public health need.

FDASIA, as a new provision, requires BPCA for paediatric drug studies to include a rationale for not including neonatal studies if none are requested. This is in line with FDA's position, prior to FDASIA, of routinely ensuring, through the PeRC, that all WRs address neonates. This new approach has identified important scientific challenges in the development of neonatal clinical trials as experience remains sparse and implementation complex.

The FDASIA somewhat reinforces the BCPA, and the FDA is monitoring precisely the impact of these changes. In the status report to the Congress in 2016, FDA noted that the few sponsors who declined the WR mentioned the following reasons:

- Product is no longer being marketed.
- Sponsor disagreed with the requirements of WR and did not believe it warranted the expenditure of further business resources.
- Sponsor would not be able to complete the studies before the due date.
- Sponsor could not complete studies before the expiration of patent or exclusivity.

(https://www.fda.gov/downloads/scienceresearch/specialtopics/pediatrictherapeuticsresearch/ucm509815.pdf)

FDA decides whether labelling changes are warranted following the results of the studies conducted under BPCA. For products granted paediatric exclusivity and receiving a paediatric labelling change, FDASIA requires FDA to post the medical, statistical, and clinical pharmacology reviews and corresponding written requests on the FDA website. This is a critical point as it emphasises the importance of making data publicly available. In another chapter, we will discuss and illustrate why publishing paediatric data is of paramount importance.

BPCA may also apply for 'off-patent' drugs; indeed, in response to the need for paediatric studies with many 'off-patent' drugs, the reauthorisation of the paediatric exclusivity incentive in BPCA included a mechanism to address such studies. Under its provisions, FDA and the National Institute of Health jointly develop a prioritised list of 'off-patent' drugs for which FDA believes paediatric studies are needed. This list is published annually in the Federal Register. FDA can issue WRs for these drugs under the usual process. If the sponsor declines the WR, FDA can refer the WR to the National Institute for Child Health and Human Development at the National Institute of Health.

FDA encourages early interactions and dialogue on paediatric development. Discussion may begin at the end-of-phase 1 (EOP1) meetings or as early as the pre-IND stage, particularly for products intended to treat life-threatening or severely debilitating illnesses. For development programs subject to PREA, these interactions should occur before the submission of the initial PSP.

3.3.2 US paediatric voucher

The term 'paediatric voucher' is incorrect but easier to understand than 'priority review voucher program'. This US priority review voucher program was created in 2007 based on a 2006 Health Affairs paper by Ridley, Grabowski, and Moe called 'Developing Drugs for Developing Countries'. Their thought process was quite innovative: 'Infectious and parasitic diseases create enormous health burdens, but because most of the people suffering from these diseases are poor, little is invested in developing treatments. We propose that developers of treatments for neglected diseases receive a "priority review voucher". The voucher could save an average of 1 year of U.S. Food and Drug Administration (FDA) review and be sold by the developer to the manufacturer of a blockbuster drug. In a well-functioning market, the voucher would speed access to highly valued treatments. Thus, the voucher could benefit consumers in both developing and developed countries at relatively low cost to the taxpayer' (Ridley et al., 2006).

Under this program, a sponsor who receives an approval for a drug or biologic for a 'rare paediatric disease' may qualify for a voucher that can be redeemed to receive a priority review of a subsequent marketing application for a different product.

On 30 September 2016, the Advancing Hope Act of 2016 (Public Law No: 114-229) amended Section 529 of the FD&C Act. Among the changes, the term 'rare paediatric disease' now means a disease that meets each of the following criteria:

1. The disease is a serious or life-threatening disease in which the serious or life-threatening manifestations primarily affect individuals aged from birth to 18 years, including age groups often called neonates, infants, children, and adolescents.
2. The disease is rare disease or conditions, within the meaning of Section 526.

The Act changed the language of Subsection (A) from, 'The disease primarily affects individuals aged from birth to 18 years, including age groups often called neonates, infants, children, and adolescents'. The full text of the Advancing Hope Act is available at https://www.gpo.gov/fdsys/pkg/BILLS-114s1878enr/pdf/BILLS-114s1878enr.pdf

Effective 90 days after the enactment of the Advancing Hope Act of 2016, the sponsor of a rare paediatric disease product application that intends to request a priority review voucher must submit such request in a cover letter to their NDA/BLA submission.

On 17 November 2014, FDA issued a draft guidance titled *Rare Paediatric Disease Priority Review Vouchers Draft Guidance for Industry*. Although this guidance does not reflect changes made to the law by the Advancing Hope Act of 2016, the guidance contains relevant information pertaining to the parts of the law not changed by the 2016 Act. Specifically, this guidance explains how FDA plans to implement Section 529 of the FD&C Act, including the process by which sponsors who are interested in receiving rare paediatric disease priority review vouchers may first request designation of their drug or biological product ('drug') as a drug for a 'rare paediatric disease'. While such designation is not required to receive a voucher, requesting this in advance will expedite a sponsor's future request for a priority review voucher.

Under the law, following approval by the Food and Drug Administration (FDA) of a treatment for a neglected or rare paediatric disease, the developer receives a voucher for priority review for a different drug. Two drugs receive priority review for each voucher: the drug winning a voucher for a neglected or rare paediatric disease and the drug using a voucher for another indication.

https://www.fda.gov/industry/developing-products-rare-diseases-conditions/rare-pediatric-disease-rpd-designation-program

The voucher may be sold. For example, a small company might win a voucher for developing a drug for a neglected disease and sell the voucher to a large company for use on a commercial disease.

This exciting initiative is not part of the FDASIA Paediatric Regulation, but it is an important initiative to stimulate paediatric development, and we wanted to mention it in this regulatory chapter as it shows the need to continue looking on how to best foster paediatric research.

3.3.3 Key features of the EU paediatric regulation

The 2006 EU Paediatric Regulation (EC) No. 1901/2006 came into force in January 2007.

The main change in the European Regulatory landscape was that all MAA for new medicines, including orphan medicines, need to contain the results of all studies and information required in a previously agreed paediatric investigation plan (PIP), unless a deferral or waiver is granted prior to the MAA submission, that is, paediatric development became mandatory.

Further to clear obligations, the Regulation introduced rewards for companies to develop medicines for use in children (see the next chapter for an in-depth assessment of the incentives).

The requirements for paediatric studies in relation to a new MAA have been applied since July 2008. For a new indication, new pharmaceutical form or new route of administration for medicines still covered by patent protection, the requirements have been applied since January 2009.

In summary, a PIP

- is a development plan aimed at ensuring that the necessary data to get a potential paediatric indication are obtained through studies;
- includes details of the timing and the measures proposed to demonstrate quality, safety, and efficacy in the paediatric population;
- describes any measures to adapt formulation for any subsets of the paediatric population (for more information on age classifications, see the ICH E11 earlier).
- must be agreed upon by the EMA's Paediatric Committee (PDCO), who can also request amendments;
- is legally binding (once agreed by PDCO) for the company and the EMA when submitting a new MAA, extension, or type II variation (e.g. new indication, formulation, route of administration).

Compliance to an agreed PIP is of paramount importance as a MAA cannot be validated in the EU before the applicant is deemed compliant with the agreed PIP.

The 2014 revised guideline on the format and content of applications for the agreement or modification of a PIP and requests for waivers or deferrals and concerning the operation of the compliance check and on the criteria for assessing significant studies brought some overall simplification, additional clarity for the compliance check, and introduced more flexibility into the application process. Additionally, extrapolation and modelling are better recognised.

3.3.3.1 Indication versus condition

The EU regulation introduced the dichotomy between indication and condition that created some confusion among pharmaceutical companies accustomed to the concept of indication used by the US regulation. While the PREA mandates the paediatric development in the same indication than in adults and the BPCA opens to additional indications than the ones pursued for the adult development, the EU regulation follows a different approach, that is, requiring a paediatric development program in the 'conditions in which a medicinal product may be authorised to treat the paediatric population'. As this introduced a key difference with this US approach, it became obvious that a systematic and consistent approach was needed to help applicants determining the paediatric condition(s) of a PIP in relation to the proposed adult indication(s). Therefore in 2012 the EMA published a policy aiming to provide guidance based on the characteristics of the product, and hierarchical classification of diseases and conditions should provide a framework for both the applicants and the PDCO evaluating the PIPs. It is interesting to cite the precise wording of the guideline (https://www.ema.europa.eu/en/documents/other/policy-determination-conditions-paediatric-investigation-plan-pip/waiver-scope-pip/waiver_en.pdf): 'Article 11 (NB: of the EU regulation) specifies the grounds for waivers of the paediatric development and refers to "condition or diseases" and to the possibility to waive specific indications, while in article 8, the Paediatric Regulation mentions "indications" in respect of existing (authorised) and new indications. However, the Paediatric Regulation does not define what a potential paediatric use is, nor does it define this potential paediatric use in relation to the indication proposed by pharmaceutical companies, which is generally but not always an adult indication. The European Commission Guideline 2008/C 243/01 provides definitions of a condition, a PIP indication and a therapeutic indication. A condition is "any deviation(s) from the normal structure or function of the body, as manifested by a characteristic set of signs and symptoms (typically a recognised distinct disease or a syndrome)" (section 1). However, this definition does not provide the link with the proposed indication. In the European Union, it is common for marketing authorisation applicants to request (and/or to be granted) a restricted indication in adults (e.g. "second-line treatment of hypertension in adults") (p 7, section 4.1] However, when submitting an application for a PIP or a waiver, the applicant is requested to specify the condition(s) corresponding to the indication(s) that will be proposed at the time of marketing authorisation. The Paediatric Committee of the EMA (PDCO) does have to assess the potential paediatric use in relation to the proposed adult indication, so the need for the definition of a systematic and predictable approach has been identified. Restricting the scope of the PIP to the proposed indication in adults would ignore potential unmet needs and paediatric use based on the properties of the medicine. This was confirmed by the Court of Justice in its judgment, stating that the proposed indication is only the starting point for the PDCO, which can go on looking at the potential use for children. It is crucial for both the PDCO and the applicants to know what the condition of reference for the potential paediatric use will be. There is a need for a balanced approach between, on the one hand keeping the possibility for the PDCO to address potential paediatric use and unmet paediatric needs, and on the other hand, requiring extensive development in children with a wide scope for the PIP. The experience gathered in the PDCO shows that the balancing exercise is complex and would benefit from some terms of reference'.

By using such long citation of the EMA guideline, we would like to stress the importance of setting up a simple and common workable frame as otherwise in our experience; it can create confusion among researchers or pharmaceutical industry.

In order to illustrate this complex question concretely, we will be using the example of Alzheimer's disease (AD) the most frequent aetiology of dementia. If dementia may occur in childhood, principally caused by lysosomal storage diseases (that are a heterogeneous group of more than 50 inherited disorders characterised by the accumulation of undigested or partially digested macromolecules causing cellular dysfunction resulting in clinical symptoms), namely, Niemann–Pick disease and Sanfilippo syndrome, the pathophysiology of these early forms of dementia is different from Alzheimer's disease, and AD simply does not exist in paediatric patients. Despite significant research in the field of AD, no significant breakthrough occurred in the past decades, and there is an urgent need to develop more research including clinical research. Neuropsychiatric symptoms (NPSs) of AD, that is, psychotic symptoms, agitation, apathy, depression, and sleep disturbances, have been recently under renewed interest, and in May 2016, the Alzheimer's Association Research Roundtable, a consortium of experts from academia, industry, and regulatory agencies revisited the topic, bringing together experts in the field to advance therapy development through a more comprehensive understanding of underlying mechanisms and application of novel clinical trial approaches (Lanctôt et al., 2017). Basically, these symptoms are among the earliest signs of neurocognitive disorders and incipient cognitive decline,

Table 3.6 NPS in Alzheimer's: potential paediatric development?

PREA – US	BPCA – US	PIP – EU
No requirement – waiver PREA requires development in the same indication than the adult indication, that is, psychotic symptoms, agitation, depression, or sleep disturbances in AD	Possible paediatric written request BPCA may trigger a PWR if the product could be used in paediatric patients as psychotic symptoms, agitation, depression, or sleep disturbances, are commonly seen in child and adolescent psychiatry	PIP or waiver The EMA policy provides the framework for identifying the condition to be considered in a PIP or waiver The elements to be considered in determining a PIP condition are as follows: – the adult indication(s) under development, – the mechanism of action (MoA) – the unmet paediatric needs – the use of an independent hierarchical classification of diseases/conditions (i.e. MedDRA – cf. definition in the succeeding text) – and whether the product is intended in this case for treatment or prevention of psychotic symptoms, agitation, depression, or sleep disturbances These elements will be considered in the previous order to identify an overarching condition A waiver will be given in this case if – the product is likely to be ineffective or unsafe (for instance due to its MoA), – or does not represent a significant therapeutic benefit over existing paediatric treatments

yet underrecognised despite causing substantial distress for both people with AD and their caregivers and contributing to early institutionalisation. NPSs are also often challenging to treat, and more clinical studies are anticipated in the future.

NPSs, with the exception of apathy, offer a perfect example to understand the difference between the EU and the US regulations and the distinction between condition and indication.

If a pharmaceutical company develops a product for psychotic symptoms, agitation, depression, or sleep disturbances, the way the EU and US regulation will evidence a definite difference (Table 3.6).

The Medical Dictionary for Regulatory Activities or MedDRA (https://www.meddra.org/how-to-use/support-documentation/english) was developed in the late 1990s, by the ICH, in order to provide 'a rich and highly specific standardised medical terminology to facilitate sharing of regulatory information internationally for medical products used by humans'. MedDRA is available and maintained in numerous languages in addition to its original English version (i.e. in Japanese, Chinese, Czech, Dutch, French, German, Hungarian, Italian, Portuguese, Russian, and Spanish). It is widely known for its use in monitory the safety monitoring of medical products during their development and after their commercialisation, but it is also used in the registration process of these products. MedDRA covers pharmaceuticals, biologics, vaccines, and drug–device combination products. 'Multiple languages allow a wide number of users to operate in their native language which promotes accuracy and precision in assigning codes. This interoperability is very powerful and allows easy sharing of data internationally… Today, its growing use worldwide by regulatory authorities, pharmaceutical companies, clinical research organisations and health care professionals allows better global protection of patient health'. MedDRA is available without charge to all regulators worldwide; academics and health care providers can also access MedDRA through the ICH MedDRA Maintenance and Support Services Organisation (MSSO). Paid subscriptions are required for pharmaceutical companies.

3.3.3.2 Waivers and deferrals

A full or partial PIP waiver can be considered for some or all subsets of the paediatric population if

- the disease or condition occurs only in adult populations, for instance, Alzheimer's disease.
- the product is likely to be ineffective or unsafe in the paediatric population or some subsets according to the ICH E11 age groups. In the field of child and adolescent psychopharmacology, actually, only the two subsets of children and adolescents are concerned by current developments in psychopharmacology. This could potentially change in the case of early preventive therapeutic interventions, like gene therapy (unfortunately, there is no indication that gene therapy can be applied in child and adolescent psychiatry in a very near future).
- the product does not represent a significant therapeutic benefit over existing treatments in children and adolescents.

In accordance with the Paediatric Regulation, the PDCO has adopted a list of conditions that occur only in adult populations. All classes of medicinal products that intended to treat these conditions will, therefore, be exempted from the requirement for a PIP (designed as 'class waivers'). The consolidated EMA decision on the list of class waivers, first adopted in 2011, has been revised, and a final new version was released on 23 July 2015 and is found at the EMA website (https://www.ema.europa.eu/en/documents/other/european-medicines-agency-decision-cw-0001-2015-23-july-2015-class-waivers-accordance-regulation-ec_en.pdf).

Deferrals of either start or completion of some or all studies in the PIP must be justified on scientific or technical or public health grounds. A deferral means an agreement to have at least one study/measure of the PIP initiated or completed after submission of the MAA in adults but

- a deferral does not exempt the applicant from submitting a full PIP,
- a deferral does not necessarily allow the applicant to defer all measures.

Deferrals can be full (concerns all the measures in the PIP) or partial (some studies may need to be started/completed at MAA submission).
A deferral will be granted when

- it is appropriate to conduct studies in adults prior to initiating studies in children,
- studies in the paediatric population will take longer to conduct than studies in adults,
- additional nonclinical data are considered necessary,
- major quality problems prevent the development of the relevant paediatric formulation.

The PDCO may refuse deferrals on the following grounds:

- Condition is predominantly/exclusively affecting children (meaning that there is a major medical need and a potential risk of off-label use).
- Serious or life-threatening conditions occurring in both adult and paediatric population for which there are currently no or limited therapeutic alternatives.

The PIP is subject to formal approval by the PDCO and must contain a comprehensive proposal of all the studies (and their timings) necessary to support the paediatric use of an individual product and cover all of the paediatric age groups and all necessary age-appropriate formulations.

Once the PDCO approves a PIP, the company will have to ensure that the paediatric development plan follows the PIP binding elements, and once the plan has been completed, the EMA will check that all studies and measures required have been performed.

Pharmaceutical companies must submit an annual report to the EMA on the progress of the PIP until all studies have been concluded.

When a company submits an application for a marketing authorisation, a new indication, new route of administration or, new formulation, the EMA will only validate the application if the company is in compliance with all measures agreed in the PIP. To facilitate the validation, the applicant can apply for a PIP compliance check with PDCO prior to submitting the application. Where the PDCO has granted a full waiver or deferral of all studies (including nonclinical studies), the applicant should include the EMA decision letter for full waiver or deferral in the application for the marketing authorisation in order to fulfil the Paediatric Regulation requirement, and a compliance check will not be necessary.

In order to avoid delays in relation to the MAA submission and review procedure, it is essential that the PIP is submitted to the EMA relatively early in the development process. The key consideration is to ensure that the MAA is not delayed. Internal preparation must, therefore, allow time for PIP process and PDCO compliance check (if applicable), all of which need to be finalised before the MAA submission.

Since June 2015, a new initiative enables free-of-charge early paediatric interaction meetings between the EMA and the sponsors to stimulate early dialogue on the paediatric development and the content and timing of PIP applications to enable timely integration of the paediatric development into the adult program. Also a more technical presubmission meeting can be obtained a few months before applying for a PIP or waiver, to ensure a smooth validation process at the time of the application.

3.3.3.3 Paediatric use marketing authorisation

The EU regulation created a voluntary path for paediatric studies in off-patent medicines called paediatric use marketing authorisation (PUMA). In this case, a sponsor, not necessarily a pharmaceutical company, can apply for a marketing authorisation that covers the indication and appropriate formulation for the paediatric population. A PUMA will benefit from 10 years of data and market protection as a reward for the development of this medicine in children. Preparation, submission, and review of a PIP relating to a PUMA application follow the same procedures as a PIP for an 'on-patent' medicine. By the end of 2017, seven PUMAs have been granted demonstrating a lack of success of this regulatory path. The reason for such a striking situation is complicated and will be discussed in the next chapter.

3.3.4 Global paediatric development

We would like to refer our readers to the comprehensive and elegant article written by key EMA and FDA authors in 2017: 'An Overview and Comparison of Regulatory Processes in the European Union and United States' (Penkov et al., 2017). If these authors use the classical disclaimer that 'the views expressed in this article are the personal views of the author(s) and may not be understood or quoted as being made on behalf of or reflecting the position of EMA or one of its committees or working parties, or FDA', they definitively present an in-depth review of the EU and US paediatric regulations, clarifying similarities and differences. Furthermore, this publication is an open-access article, enabling to a wider distribution, illustrating the importance of access to paediatric publications that we will discuss in another chapter of this book (Why do we need to publish paediatric data?). In the succeeding text, we use (and slightly modified) the Appendix A of their 2017 publication: 'Summary Table of Similarities and Differences Between Current EU and US Legislation'.

	FDA BPCA/ FDASIA 2012	FDA PREA/ FDASIA 2012	EU EMA Regulation 2007
Applies to	Incentive	Requirement	Incentive and requirement
Scope of paediatric development	Any indication in the paediatric population where there is potential for therapeutic benefit	Same as adult indication	Derived from adult indication, within same condition
Types of products	All medicinal products	New products and biosimilars	New products; authorised products under patent/SPC if applying for new indication/route/form
Orphan-designated excluded?	No	Yes	No

Continued

	FDA BPCA/ FDASIA 2012	FDA PREA/ FDASIA 2012	EU EMA Regulation 2007
Paediatric development	Optional	Mandatory unless waived	Mandatory unless waived
Instrument	Written response	PSP	PIP
Submission fees	No	No; however, reports submitted as a NDA/BLA or sNDA (fees apply)	No
Waiver	NA	Four grounds	Three grounds
Timing of plan submission	Anytime	EOP2 in adults	EOP1 in adults (during phase 2 if justified)
Main reward	Six-month add-on exclusivity	None	Six-month SPC extension; 2 years for orphan-designated products
Decision	FDA review division (PeRC advisory)	Review division (PeRC advisory)	EMA after opinion from PDCO
Scientific advice	Normally included in global licensing fee	Normally included in global licensing fee	Free for paediatric development
PAC[a]	Yes	Yes	No

[a] For studies conducted under BPCA or PREA, the US legislation also requires a paediatric-focused safety review by the Paediatric Advisory Committee (PAC) 18 months after FDA approves a labeling change.

The FDA Paediatric Advisory Committee advises and makes recommendations to the Commissioner of Food and Drugs regarding the following:

- Paediatric research
- Identification of research priorities related to paediatric therapeutics and the need for additional treatments of specific paediatric diseases or conditions
- Ethics, design, and analysis of clinical trials related to paediatric medicinal products
- Paediatric labelling disputes
- Adverse event reports for drugs granted paediatric exclusivity and any safety issues that may occur
- Any other paediatric issue or paediatric labelling dispute involving FDA-regulated products
- Research involving children as subjects
- Any other matter involving paediatrics for which FDA has regulatory responsibility

3.3.4.1 Facilitating integrated paediatric development in EU and US

Since 2007, EMA and FDA have established monthly teleconferences to discuss product-specific paediatric development and topics under the terms of confidentiality agreement. The objective of these exchanges is to facilitate an integrated paediatric development across the two regions, to enhance the paediatric knowledge of clinical trials and to avoid exposing children to unnecessary trials. Japan's PMDA, Health Canada, and Australia's Therapeutic Goods Administration are also part of these teleconferences, creating a genuine Paediatric Cluster.

The monthly discussions include ethical, safety, and paediatric study feasibility issues as well as protocol discussions. The type of information exchanged includes the following:

- PIPs
- WRs
- PDCO discussions
- Waivers (full and partial) and deferrals
- Choice of comparator and efficacy endpoints
- Status of ongoing paediatric studies
- Results of paediatric studies
- Safety concerns, including clinical holds
- Plans for long-term safety monitoring
- Topics related to product classes (e.g. safety concerns and general study approaches

EMA and FDA have also discussed piloting joint early paediatric interactions with sponsors to further support global paediatric product development (before submission of PIP, PSP, and PPSR).

3.3.5 Global paediatric development strategy

Paediatric development has always been challenging for all actors including the pharmaceutical industry. Currently, one major challenge for pharmaceutical companies is to get a viable paediatric strategy that encompasses the different paediatric regulations requirements in term of scope and timing of the paediatric development. Paediatric development should not be performed 'just' because US and EU regulations mandate it; paediatric development should follow a clear strategy that not simply reflects a company commitment to follow the regulation but that demonstrates a true 'paediatric ambition'.

Therefore, it is of paramount importance to aim for early and potentially frequent interactions with authorities, develop scientifically and ethically sound paediatric programmes and propose optimal submission and realistic completion timelines. I was actually shocked a few years ago hearing European Regulators referring to amazing reasons to not performed a PIP, like 'insomnia not occurring in children' (sic).

We are not in this chapter going into details of contents and timelines of paediatric development plans, just giving essential information, as the details can be found on the EMA and FDA websites and the precise strategy will always only be project specific.

We want to emphasise that contents and timelines should always reflect a clear ambition and willingness to bring better medicines for children.

Finally, we would also like to stress the numerous opportunities of interactions with the regulators, including early interactions, that both US and EU regulations offer. The experiences shared by all the authors of this book are unanimous; constructive dialogue with regulators both in EU and United States enables us to find common grounds and understanding for better paediatric development.

3.3.5.1 Contents of paediatric developments: PSP, PWR, PPSR, and PIPs

	FDA – BPCA Proposed Paediatric Study Request (PPSR)/ Written Request (WR) 2012	FDA – PREA Paediatric Study Plan (PSP) 2012	EU – Paediatric Investigational Plan (PIP) 2007
Template/content	PPSR template pertaining to rationale for studies; study design; and formulations FDA will use the PPSR to draft the Written Request	Up to 60 pages Overview of disease/ product, outline/ plans of paediatric studies (clinical and nonclinical), background supporting data (adult), waiver/ deferral requests, formulation, timelines, agreements with other regulatory authorities	Should be a maximum 40 pages Administrative and product information; Info on disease and therapeutic benefit; Application for a waiver if applicable; Proposed paediatric development plan; Request for deferral if applicable. *More background info on drug/adult program may be needed; often first contact with EMA*
Guidance	Draft 1999 guidance 'Guidance for industry: qualifying for paediatric exclusivity under Section 505A of the Federal Food, Drug, and Cosmetic Act' Advice on FDA website	PSP (PREA) Draft 2016 guidance – 'Content of and Process for Submitting Initial Paediatric Study Plans and Amended Initial Paediatric Study Plans' Advice on FDA website	EU guideline – European Commission Guideline regarding the format and content of PIP and waiver applications Advice on the EMA website

3.3.5.2 Timing of paediatric development plan submission in US and EU

	FDA BPCA/ FDASIA 2012	FDA PREA/ FDASIA 2012	EU EMA Regulation 2007
Timing of plan submission	Anytime	EOP2 in adults	EOP1 in adults (during phase 2 if justified)

3.3.6 Review PIP procedures and timelines

The PDCO review procedure takes a maximum of 120 days of active review, separated by a clock stop if needed.

For a full waiver request, the PDCO shall within 60 days without clock stop adopt an opinion as to whether or not a product-specific waiver should be granted (Fig. 3.2).

3.3.7 PSP review procedures and timelines

The initial PSP should be submitted within 60 days of end-of-phase 2 meeting or in case of the absence of a meeting before the initiation of the phase 3 programme. The total review and approval time of the PSP is 210 days (Fig. 3.3).

3.3.8 Review and timelines PPSR – PWR

There is no specific timeframe for FDA action on a PPSR, and estimations vary among reviewing divisions, with an industry average of 120 days.

Once the FDA receives a PPSR, the Review Division in collaboration with the PeRC will review the PPSR and provide comments back to the sponsor. There may be multiple iterations of the PPSR before issuance of a WR.

The review divisions have primary responsibility for drafting WRs. After a WR is issued to the sponsor, the sponsor has 180 days to respond, accepting or declining.

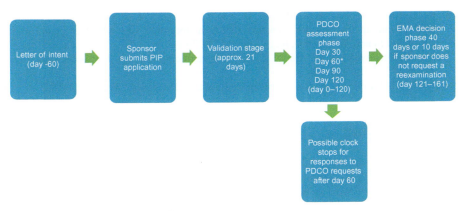

Fig. 3.2 PIP procedures and timelines.

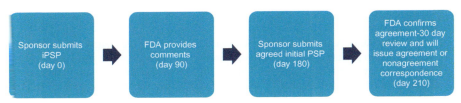

Fig. 3.3 PSP procedures and timelines.

3.3.9 Conclusion

In my clinical experience, spending a full year as a consultation-liaison psychiatrist in different paediatric units among a paediatric university hospital, I was always amazed by what the kids were telling me, and I want to share the vivid memory of one of my young patients who 1 day gave me a real-life lesson and the best genuine definition of altruism: 'You know, I am not sure that the new treatment they are giving me will help me, but if it can help my friends (pointing towards the other rooms), I would be very happy'.

These young patients and their families made me understand what paediatric regulations are standing for and consequently mean, and we hope that this chapter will give enough insights to understand the worldwide paediatric regulations and how to optimally work with them not to comply to a processes but to convey a genuine paediatric ambition.

References

Auby, P., 2014. The European Union Pediatric legislation: impact on pharmaceutical research in pediatric populations. Clin. Invest. 4 (11), 1013–1019.

Lanctôt, K.L., Amatniek, J., Ancoli-Israel, S., Arnold, S.E., Ballard, C., Cohen-Mansfield, J., Ismail, Z., Lyketsos, C., Miller, D.S., Musiek, E., Osorio, R.S., Rosenberg, P.B., Satlin, A., Steffens, D., Tariot, P., Bain, L.J., Carrillo, M.C., Hendrix, J.A., Jurgens, H., Boot, B., 2017. Neuropsychiatric signs and symptoms of Alzheimer's disease: new treatment paradigms. Alzheimers Dement. 3 (3), 440–449.

Penkov, D., Tomasi, P., Eichler, I., Murphy, D., Yao, L.P., Temeck, J., 2017. Pediatric medicine development: an overview and comparison of regulatory processes in the European Union and United States. Ther. Innov. Regul. Sci. 51 (3), 360–371.

Ridley, D.B., Grabowski, H.G., Moe, J.L., 2006. Developing drugs for developing countries. Health Aff. 25 (2), 313–324.

Shirkey, H., 1999. Editorial comment: therapeutic orphans. Pediatrics 104 (3), 583–584.

Further reading

EC, 2002. Better Medicines for Children. Proposed Regulatory Actions on Paediatric Medicinal Products. Consultation Document. http://ec.europa.eu/health/files/pharmacos/docs/doc2002/.

https://www.ema.europa.eu/en/documents/other/european-medicines-agency-decision-cw-0001-2015-23-july-2015-class-waivers-accordance-regulation-ec_en.pdf.

https://www.ich.org/home.html.

https://www.meddra.org/how-to-use/support-documentation/english.

National Vaccine Injury Compensation Program (VICP), 1988. www.hrsa.gov/vaccinecompensation/index.html.

Rivera, D.R., Hartzema, A.G., 2014. Pediatric exclusivity: evolving legislation and novel complexities within pediatric therapeutic development. Ann. Pharmacother. 48 (3), 369–379.

US FDA Safety and Innovation Act (FDASIA), 2012. www.fda.gov/RegulatoryInformation/Legislation/FederalFoodDrugandCosmeticActDCAct/SignificantAmendmentstotheFDCAct/FDASIA.

www.who.int/childmedicines/en.

Are the paediatric rewards adapted?[☆]

Geneviève Michaux[a], Beatrice Stirner[b]
[a]Mayer Brown LLP, Brussels, Belgium, [b]Swiss Federal Institute of Intellectual Property, Bern, Switzerland

On 12 December 2006, the European legislature adopted the Paediatric Regulation[a] after several years of heated debates. The purpose of the new legislation is to generate data on the safety and efficacy of medicinal products when used in children and to promote the development of paediatric medicinal products. The European paediatric regime is based on a stick-carrot philosophy and thus contains two main parts. The first part concerns the paediatric obligation and procedure. Experience had showed that pharmaceutical companies do not voluntarily invest in paediatric research; hence, they had to be forced to conduct paediatric studies. The second part concerns the rewards granted for having fulfilled the paediatric obligation.

In a nutshell, the 'paediatric obligation' can be described as follows: marketing authorisation applications (MAA) and applications for a new therapeutic indication (type II variation) or a new pharmaceutical form or route of administration (line extension) of a medicinal product that is protected by a supplementary protection certificate (SPC)[b] or a patent that qualifies for an SPC, must contain the paediatric data generated by the implementation of a paediatric investigation plan (PIP) proposed by the company before Phase II and agreed upon by European Medicines Agency (EMA), unless a waiver or a deferral has been granted by the EMA for certain studies included in the PIP. The Paediatric Regulation contains other obligations, but its primary objective is to impose the paediatric obligation, to set forth the paediatric procedure, (that is, the procedure for the approval of PIPs, waivers, and deferrals), and to create the Paediatric Committee (PDCO), a new scientific committee within the EMA.

Subject to certain conditions being met, the fulfilment of the paediatric obligation leads to a reward, which depends on the nature and status of the medicinal product.

[☆] The views and opinions expressed in this article are those of the author and do not necessarily reflect the views, opinions, or position of the Swiss Federal Institute of Intellectual Property.
[a] Regulation (EC) No. 1901/2006 of the European Parliament and of the Council of 12 December 2006 on medicinal products for paediatric use and amending regulation (EEC) No. 1768/92, Directive 2001/20/EC, Directive 2001/83/EC and Regulation (EC) No. 726/2004.
[b] Regulation (EC) No. 469/2009 of the European Parliament and of the Council of 6 May 2009 concerning the supplementary protection certificate for medicinal products. It has codified and replaced Council Regulation (EEC) No. 1768/92 of 18 June 1992 concerning the creation of a supplementary protection certificate for medicinal products.

The Paediatric Regulation institutes three rewards: the so-called 'SPC extension', the 'market exclusivity extension', and the paediatric-use marketing authorisation (PUMA).

This contribution focuses on paediatric rewards. We refer to the previous chapter, Worldwide Paediatric Regulations, for detailed explanations on the paediatric obligation and procedure.

Given the complexity of the Paediatric Regulation, we first provide a few explanations on the scope of the Paediatric Regulation. Furthermore, the paediatric rewards relate to existing protections; hence, we also briefly explain those protections before diving into the intricacies of the paediatric rewards.

Paediatric rewards are mainly governed by Articles 36 and 52 (SPC extension), Article 37 (market exclusivity extension), and Article 30 (PUMA) of the Paediatric Regulation. Like many other articles of the Paediatric Regulation, these legal provisions are vague, thus giving rise to many issues. To date, the European Commission has not published a guideline on paediatric rewards. Several national patent offices (NPO), however, have included advice on SPC extensions in their official guidelines on SPC, and courts have been asked to rule on certain questions.

By the end of 2017, around 50 SPC extensions, 7 market exclusivity extensions, and 7 PUMAs had been granted, and many of them had only been awarded recently. The reason for such a striking situation is complex. According to the European Commission and the EMA, paediatric rewards only started being granted after several years because PIPs first had to be completed and long deferrals had been accepted. Indeed, most PIPs include and have included (long) deferrals, which prevent companies from collecting the rewards. The need for long deferrals, however, was and is due to the EMA being very demanding with regard to the need for paediatric studies, including the number and the features of those studies (number of patients, endpoints, etc.). To date, many PIPs are still ongoing that will hopefully trigger paediatric rewards soon and restore, albeit slightly, the unbalance between PIPs and paediatric rewards.

A more important question is whether the rewards are adapted to their objective, which is to compensate for mandatory paediatric development. The answer can partly be found in the report prepared by the European Commission ('Commission') after 10 years of application of the Paediatric Regulation.[c] Another part of the answer should result from the Commission's ongoing studies on the combined effect of the Paediatric Regulation and the Orphan Regulation.[d] Four points, however, are already established before the Commission collects all the relevant data and information: the costs of paediatric development is, on average, five times higher than initially expected; the PUMA is a failure; obtaining a reward for orphan medicinal products is more challenging than for any other category of medicinal products; and paediatric development of new medicinal products without patent protection or orphan designation (such as vaccines) is not rewarded at all. Hopefully, the Commission will fix those issues.

---

[c] Regulation (EC) No. 141/2000 of the European Parliament and of the Council of 16 December 1999 on orphan medicinal products.
[d] European Commission, https://ec.europa.eu/info/law/better-regulation/initiatives/ares-2017-6059807_en.

The last chapter will introduce the Swiss incentive system for the development of paediatric medicinal products. The new Swiss legislation entered into force on 1 January 2019. This chapter will provide an overview of the Swiss measures, which vary from the EU measures, and of the implementation of the new legislation, including the revised Patents Act and the Therapeutic Products Act.

4.1 Scope of application of the paediatric obligation

MAA for new medicinal products and applications for a new therapeutic indication (type II variation), a new pharmaceutical form or route of administration (line extension) of a medicinal product that is protected by a SPC, or a patent that qualifies for an SPC, must contain the paediatric data generated by the implementation of a PIP agreed upon by EMA, unless a waiver or a deferral has been agreed by the EMA for certain studies included in the PIP.

The paediatric obligation refers to the mandatory submission of paediatric data with a MAA or an application for a type II variation (new indications) or a line extension (new pharmaceutical form or route of administration) (collectively 'regulatory applications'). In those cases, the PIP is also mandatory, but it remains only a tool designed to generate the paediatric data that will be required at the time of the regulatory application.

4.1.1 Mandatory paediatric obligation (Art. 7 and Art. 8)

While the Paediatric Regulation applies to all medicinal products for human use, the paediatric obligation only applies to (i) MAA for new medicinal products ('new medicinal products'—Art. 7) and (ii) applications for new therapeutic indications, new pharmaceutical forms, and/or new routes of administration of medicinal products that are both already approved and still protected by a SPC or by a patent that qualifies for an SPC ('approved/on-patent medicinal products'—Art. 8).

The paediatric obligation does not apply to applications for other variations or line extensions of approved/on-patent medicinal products or to applications for approved medicinal products that are not or no longer protected by an SPC or a patent that qualifies for an SPC ('approved/off-patent medicinal products'). For the latter category of medicinal products, the paediatric obligation is voluntary—see the succeeding text. Moreover, certain categories of medicinal products are exempted from the obligation—see the succeeding text.

The distinction between those three categories of medicinal products—new, approved/on-patent, and approved/off-patent—is central to the Paediatric Regulation.

The wording of Articles 7 and 8 of the Paediatric Regulation is not clear and has been debated. The focus of this contribution is the rewards; hence, we will not explain the interpretations of Articles 7 and 8 adopted by the European Commission/EMA and the debates around them. We, however, stress that the concept of 'new medicinal product' is interpreted as referring to a medicinal product that contains an active substance that is new for the company.

4.1.2 Optional paediatric obligation (Art. 30)

With regard to approved/off-patent medicinal products, companies may voluntarily opt to be subject to the paediatric obligation, that is, to implement a PIP agreed upon by the EMA.

In such a case, the company may apply for and obtain a paediatric-use marketing authorisation (PUMA). PUMA is a new category of MAs that are exclusively dedicated to children (paediatric indication and paediatric form).

While the voluntary fulfilment of the paediatric obligation also leads to a reward, this reward is not such as to create a real incentive, at least for innovative companies. This probably explains why the option has not been used much so far and why the Paediatric Regulation foresees community funding for paediatric research on approved/off-patent medicinal products (Art. 40).

4.1.3 Exemptions from paediatric obligation (Art. 9)

The paediatric obligation applies to all medicinal products for human use, including orphan medicinal products and advanced therapy medicinal products.

However, medicinal products to be authorised under certain legal provisions of Directive 2001/83[e] are expressly exempted from the paediatric obligation: generics, biosimilars and hybrids (Art. 10), substances with well-established medicinal use (Art. 10a), homeopathic medicinal products (Art. 13–16), and traditional herbal medicinal products (Art. 16a–16i).

Moreover, in accordance with the concept of global marketing authorisation (global MA), the EMA only requires one PIP in case of duplicate MAA, and MAA based on consent (Art. 10c) are exempted from the paediatric obligation, provided that it relates to a reference medicinal product for which a MAA was filed after 26 July 2008.

Of note, MAA for fixed dose combination medicinal products (Art. 10b) and so-called mixed MAA (Art. 8(3), Annex I) are not exempted from the paediatric obligation.

4.2 Types paediatric rewards

The fulfilment of the paediatric obligation leads to a reward, which varies depending on the nature and status of the medicinal product and is subject to stringent conditions. The Paediatric Regulation institutes three rewards—the SPC extension, the market exclusivity extension, and the PUMA—that each raises issues.

---

[e] Dir. 2001/83 Directive 2001/83/EC of the European Parliament and of the Council of 6 November 2001 on the Community code relating to medicinal products for human use.

4.2.1 Background on SPC, market exclusivity, and data exclusivity

4.2.1.1 Supplementary protection certificate

Although SPCs have been created and are governed by a European regulation, they are in essence national because they are granted by the national patent office ('NPO') of each member state, and the SPC rules are applied and interpreted at the national level.

A substance—chemical or biological—may be developed as a medicinal product, a cosmetic, a detergent, etc. If it is developed as a medicinal product, European pharmaceutical law applies, which means that specific tests are required and that a MA must be granted by a governmental authority before the medicinal product may be placed on the market. Testing and MA procedure are an important investment financially and in time as they take on average 8–12 years. During that time, the patent holder may not exploit its patent. The SPC seeks to compensate the patent holder for that loss of patent protection.

Once the substance has been developed as a medicinal product and a MA has been granted, the patent holder may ask the NPO to grant an SPC in relation to one of the patents protecting that substance (the 'basic patent'). Such application may be filed in each member state where there are a valid basic patent and a valid MA granted in accordance with EU pharmaceutical law. The application for the SPC must be filed with the NPO within 6 months of the date of the basic patent or the MA, whichever comes last.

The SPC grants the same rights and obligations as the basic patent but only for medicinal products and with a limited term. The term of the SPC is calculated on the basis of the date of filing of the patent application and the date of the first MA in the European Economic Area ('EEA'), with a maximum of 5 years.

4.2.1.2 Market exclusivity

Market exclusivity is the regulatory exclusivity granted to orphan medicinal products authorised in the European Union under the Orphan Regulation.[f]

While the SPC requires a formal approval from the NPO, market exclusivity results from the mere combination of an orphan designation and an MA. An orphan designation is granted by the Commission to active substances that are being developed for the treatment, prevention, or diagnosis of rare conditions provided that certain conditions (called 'designation criteria') are met. The medicinal product that contains that active substance and is subsequently authorised for a therapeutic indication that is part of the rare condition automatically benefits for market exclusivity.

Market exclusivity prevents the EMA and the national competent authorities from accepting another MAA or granting an MA (or a variation) for a same or similar medicinal product and for the same therapeutic indication.

Market exclusivity lasts for 10 years from the date of the MA for the orphan medicinal product. The 10-year period may be reduced to 6 years if, at the end of the fifth

---

[f] See footnote c.

year, it is established that the designation criteria are no longer met, *inter alia*, where it is shown that the medicinal product is sufficiently profitable not to justify maintenance of market exclusivity.[g] So far no market exclusivity has been reduced by the European Commission. The Commission refused to reduce the market exclusivity for Plenadren, which had been requested by the United Kingdom.

Market exclusivity does not prevent the acceptance of a MAA or the grant of a MA for a same or similar medicinal product, for the same indication if (i) the holder of the MA (MAH) for the original orphan medicinal product has given his consent; (ii) the MAH for the original orphan medicinal product is unable to supply sufficient quantities of the medicinal product; or (iii) the second applicant can establish that the second medicinal product, although similar to the orphan medicinal product already authorised is safer, more effective or otherwise clinically superior.

Commission Regulation 847/2000 provides relevant definitions, including the concept of 'similarity' that is the cornerstone of market exclusivity protection. It is for the CHMP (or the competent national authority as the second product may but need not be an orphan product) to decide whether the second product is similar and, as the case, may be clinically superior to the current orphan medicinal product for market exclusivity purposes.

Once the second applicant with a designated orphan medicinal product succeeds in obtaining an MA for their product, they share the market exclusivity with the first MAH for the remaining duration of the 10-year period granted to the first product. If the second product is not designated, it is only protected by data exclusivity but does not share market exclusivity.

4.2.1.3 Data exclusivity and marketing protection

New medicinal products, that is, medicinal products that contain a new active substance, are protected by 8-year data exclusivity followed by 2 years of marketing protection. Data exclusivity means that other companies are prevented from referring to the nonclinical and clinical data in the MA dossier in order to seek the authorisation of another, 'generic' medicinal product. Marketing protection means that the generic product authorised by reference to the MA dossier of an innovative product (called the 'reference medicinal product') may not be placed on the market.

One year is added to the marketing protection period if a new indication that is considered to bring a significant therapeutic benefit over the existing treatments, is approved during the first 8 years of protection.

Therefore, overall, a new medicinal product may benefit from $8+2+1$ years protection against generic competition.

The $8+2+1$ years protection period starts running with the global MA,[h] that is, the first MA granted for the medicinal product that contains a new active substance.

---

[g] European Commission, Guideline on aspects of the application of Article 8(2) of Regulation (EC) No. 141/2000: Review of the period of market exclusivity of orphan medicinal products, 17 Sept. 2008.

[h] On the concept of global MA, see Eudralex, Vol. 2, Chapter 1—Marketing Authorisation, (Dec. 2018). https://ec.europa.eu/health/sites/health/files/files/eudralex/vol-2/vol2a_chap1_en.pdf.

After the granting of the global MA, all subsequent authorisation falls into the global MA and no new development benefits from an additional protection (except for a new indication that is considered to bring a significant therapeutic benefit over the existing treatments).

4.2.2 Types of rewards (Art. 36–39)

The Paediatric Regulation institutes three paediatric rewards, depending on the nature and status of the medicinal product concerned.

SPC extension (Art. 36)—The reward for new medicinal products (Art. 7) and approved/on-patent medicinal products (Art. 8) is a 6-month extension of the term of the SPC ('SPC extension') unless the medicinal product has an orphan designation.

Market exclusivity extension (Art. 37)—For new medicinal products (Art. 7) and approved/on-patent medicinal products (Art. 8) with an orphan designation, the reward is two additional years of market exclusivity ('market exclusivity extension').

PUMA (Art. 30)—If a company voluntarily implements a PIP for an approved/off-patent medicinal product, it will be granted a PUMA. The reward is the PUMA because it does not fall into the global MA and thus triggers an 8-year data exclusivity followed by the 2 + 1 years marketing protection of the new paediatric data.

The second 'reward' for approved/off-patent medicinal products is the brand name. The paediatric medicinal product authorised by the PUMA may take the same brand name as the adult medicinal product despite a separate MA. The rationale is to allow the paediatric medicinal product to benefit from the investment made in the adult brand name.

4.2.3 Requirements for paediatric rewards

The Paediatric Regulation sets forth stringent requirements for being eligible and obtaining the rewards. These requirements have been made even more stringent by the Commission's interpretations.

4.2.3.1 Substantive requirements

The substantive requirements for benefiting from a paediatric reward are the following:

- The product must be approved by all Member States.
- The paediatric data must comply with the agreed PIP.
- The results of paediatric studies must be mentioned in the summary of product characteristics (SmPC).
- Significant studies must be completed after 26 January 2007.

Except for approved/off-patent medicinal products, the approval of a new paediatric indication and/or formulation is not a requirement for the reward, provided that the results of the—unsuccessful—paediatric studies are included in the SmPC. In most cases, the results of the paediatric studies are useful for healthcare professionals and thus worth being added in the SmPC of the product.

Additional requirements apply where the reward is the SPC extension:

- The product may not have an orphan designation.
- The MAH may not have obtained the additional year of marketing protection ('+1 year') for a new indication with a significant therapeutic benefit.
- No previous SPC extension has been granted.

Most of those requirements raise issues that render uncertain the grant of a reward.

4.2.3.2 Procedural requirements

Procedural requirements only apply to the SPC extension. Article 52 of the Paediatric Regulation has amended the SPC Regulation to adapt certain SPC rules to the SPC extension and include a new procedure.

4.2.4 SPC extension: Substantive and procedural requirements

The SPC extension raises many issues. SPCs and SPC extensions are granted by the NPO, not by the Commission or the EMA.

4.2.4.1 Approval of the product in all member states (Art. 36(3))

This requirement raises two issues: the meaning of the term 'product' and of the expression 'all member states'.

'Product'—The term 'product' is very vague and could be interpreted in several ways.

It could be interpreted by reference to the concept of a global MA. Such an interpretation would ensure consistency not only throughout the Paediatric Regulation but also between the Paediatric Regulation and the general pharmaceutical rules (Directive 2001/83[i] and Regulation 726/2004[j]). Moreover, it would be equitable to use the same notion for obligations (Articles 7 and 8) and rewards. It is unfair to the industry to adopt a broad interpretation when it comes to obligations, which ensures that as many products as possible are subject to the paediatric obligation, while simultaneously adopting a strict interpretation when it comes to rewards, which results *de facto* in fewer medicinal products benefiting from the rewards.

The term 'product' could also be understood by reference to the SPC Regulation. Article 8(1)(d)(ii) of the SPC Regulation (which determines the documents to be filed with the NPO for being granted an SPC extension—see the succeeding text) contains a provision identical to Article 36(3) and in the SPC Regulation, the term 'product' is legally defined as 'active substance or combination of active substances'. Such an interpretation would ensure some consistency throughout the SPC Regulation. More importantly, to the extent that the term is legally defined, another meaning may arguably not be envisaged without violating the SPC Regulation.

---

[i] See footnote e.
[j] Regulation (EC) No. 726/2004 of the European Parliament and of the Council of 31 March 2004 laying down union procedures for the authorisation and supervision of medicinal products for human and veterinary use and establishing a European Medicines Agency.

In practice, the Commission adopts the most restrictive interpretation and considers that the term 'product' refers to the *paediatric* medicinal product and thus that the company may not obtain the paediatric reward before the paediatric medicinal product is authorised by the 28 member states (and the EFTA States—see the succeeding text).

However, Article 36(3) does not contain this specification, while Article 33 does ('the product on the market taking into account the paediatric indication'), thus showing that the EU legislature knew the difference and could have used the same wording for Article 36(3).

More importantly, during the first year of application of the Paediatric Regulation, the Commission's interpretation mortgaged heavily the chances of extending the SPCs for approved medicinal products. Regulatory approval procedures take quite some time, and some member states take (much) longer than the period set by law to issue the MA. As a result, the Commission's interpretation left a company dependent on each of the 28 (30 in fact—see the succeeding text) member states recognising the company's fulfilment of its statutory obligations for obtaining the reward.

Most NPO have accepted the Commission's interpretation that the approval relates to the paediatric rather than the adult medicinal product. As a result, the period of time between the completion of the PIP and the filing of the application for SPC extension is longer (as the paediatric version has to be authorised), which may be an issue when the SPC is close to expiration.

'All member states'—Pursuant to Protocol 1 of the EEA Agreement, the expression 'all member states' only refers to the EU Member States and not to the three EFTA States (Iceland, Liechtenstein, and Norway). In light of that definition, companies should not be denied the reward because the 'product' is not approved in one of the EFTA States.

Nevertheless, the Commission considers that the requirement includes the three EFTA States since the Paediatric Regulation has been formally included in the list of EU legislations to which the EEA Agreement applies. This happened on 5 May 2017 when the EEA Joint Committee adopted Decision No. 92/2017 amending Annex II (Technical regulations, standards, testing and certification) and Annex XVII (Intellectual Property) to the EEA Agreement. The integration took more than 10 years due to an institutional disagreement between the EU and the EFTA States.

Decision No. 92/2017 of the Joint Committee incorporates into the EEA Agreement the Paediatric Regulation and the codified SPC Regulation. It provides that:

- The reference to 'all member states' does not include Liechtenstein.
- For a period of 5 years, applications for SPC extension may be filed within 6 months from expiration of the basic patent. That transitional period starts upon the entry into force of the Paediatric Regulation in the EFTA State. The SPC extension only takes effect for the time following that entry into force and the date of publication of the application for the SPC extension.
- If the SPC expires less than 7 months after the entry into force of the Paediatric Regulation in the EFTA State, the application for the SPC extension must be filed within 1 month from that entry into force. The SPC extension only takes effect for the time following the date of publication of the application for the SPC extension.
- If a third party has commercially used the invention or has made serious preparations for such use between the expiration of the SPC and the date of publication of the application for the SPC extension, it can continue using the invention.

Following the integration of the Paediatric Regulation and codified SPC Regulation into the EEA Agreement, Iceland and Norway introduced the Paediatric Regulation into their national law. The Norwegian implementing law became applicable on 1 September 2017, and the Icelandic implementing law became applicable on 1 June 2018.

4.2.4.2 Compliance with an agreed PIP (Art. 36(1))

Article 36(1) requires compliance with an agreed PIP, but Article 36(2) specifies that the inclusion of the statement referred to in Article 28(3) in an MA should be used for the purposes of applying Article 36(1). Article 28(3) refers to the compliance statement. The legal requirement, therefore, is that the MA contains a statement of compliance with the PIP agreed by the EMA.

A few years ago, there was a debate about the compliance statement for purposes of the paediatric reward. It is now commonly accepted that compliance with an agreed PIP is formalised by the compliance statement that is issued by the competent health authority and is included in the MA. The PDCO opinion on compliance is not sufficient.

Compliance with the agreed PIP is checked by the PDCO after full completion of the PIP. However, given the broad scope of the PIP as well as the number and complexity of the paediatric studies in the PIP, deferrals have been accepted for most PIP, and completion of a PIP takes several years. During that time, companies typically submit one or more regulatory applications, and the PDCO performs a so-called 'partial compliance check' each time such a regulatory application falls under the scope of the Paediatric Regulation (Articles 7 and 8).

In cases of noncompliance, either the competent national authority or the EMA does not validate the regulatory application, or the company is not eligible for a reward, depending on the stage at which noncompliance is detected.

Compliance Check—The competent authority must verify compliance with the PIP, that is, that the paediatric data submitted by the company in the regulatory application are those resulting from the specific studies/measures detailed in the PIP.

The authority in charge of assessing and deciding on compliance with the PIP is the authority in charge of granting the MA. However, both the company and the competent authority may ask the PDCO to give an opinion on compliance. The company may not file the regulatory application until the PDCO has given an opinion, and the opinion procedure may take up to 60 days.

In practice, companies require a PDCO opinion before filing their regulatory applications because this gives them an opportunity to 'fix' the PIP and become compliant. Indeed, if the PDCO concludes on noncompliance with the PIP, the company has two options: to generate the right data or to modify the PIP (so that it fits to the existing data). In cases of 'minor' noncompliance, the PDCO will generally accept a modification of the PIP in order not to delay further the approval of the paediatric medicinal product. In such a case, the regulatory procedure is delayed by 4–5 months.

The agreed PIP generally requires the company to conduct several paediatric studies that it details. Initially, the PDCO checked compliance with each detail of each study in accordance with the Commission's main guideline on PIP. In 2014, the Commission revised its guideline, which now provides that compliance check is limited to the key elements of the EMA decision on the PIP and the minimum critical elements of each measure in the PIP decision. This has made the compliance check a much more administrative process and has reduced the number of noncompliance. Furthermore, where the PIP uses conditional terms ('could') or examples ('such as'), the elements to which those refer should not be checked for compliance.

The compliance check does not concern the quality, safety, and efficacy of the active substance when used in the paediatric population. If the PDCO designs the PIP and thus determines the studies that—in its opinion—are necessary to show the safety and efficacy of the medicinal product in children, it is not involved in the scientific review of the paediatric data. This scientific assessment remains in the exclusive control of the competent regulatory authority. Therefore although the PDCO includes members of the CHMP, there is a risk of divergence between the PDCO requirements and the CHMP requirements, and in case of divergence, the PDCO does not prevail. In other words, a PIP is not a guarantee of approval of the paediatric indication.

Compliance is checked twice, once before the validation of the regulatory application and once during the scientific assessment of the paediatric data. At the time of filing of the regulatory application, the PDCO makes a full compliance check. If the paediatric data are found to be noncompliant, the regulatory application is declared invalid. If they are found to be compliant, the regulatory application can go through validation. A second compliance check is made during scientific assessment. At this stage, the competent regulatory authority thoroughly examines all the paediatric data and may discover noncompliance that was not detected at the time of filing. In such a case, the regulatory application remains valid, but the company is not eligible for the paediatric reward.

Where the competent regulatory authority concludes on compliance with the PIP, a statement of compliance is included in the MA (Art. 28(3)). In practice, the compliance statement is in an annex to the MA (centralised procedure) or in the MA decision (decentralised procedure).

Deferrals and Partial Compliance Check—The PDCO only conducts a compliance check after the PIP has been fully completed. Until then, that is, while studies are deferred, the PDCO conducts a partial compliance check each time the company submits a regulatory application that falls within the scope of the Paediatric Regulation (Article 7 or 8).

Ideally, all paediatric studies would be completed before the company submits the regulatory application for adults, and the medicinal product would be approved for adults and children at the same time. This however would delay the approval of adult indications because for ethical reasons, medicinal products are only tested in children after having been tested in adults. The Paediatric Regulation, therefore, includes the possibility for the company to request a deferral, that is, that the completion or initiation of one or more paediatric studies be postponed until after the expected date of submission of the regulatory application for adults. For more information on deferrals, see the previous chapter on Worldwide Paediatric Regulations.

In case of a deferral, the company is not eligible for the paediatric reward until all the deferred studies are completed (or initiated). A deferral thus postpones both the completion or initiation of certain or all paediatric studies and the eligibility for the paediatric reward.

The broad scope of the PIP and the EMA's demands with regard to paediatric studies result in most PIP including (long) deferrals. If compliance with the PIP were to be checked only after completion of all the studies in the PIP, regulatory applications for adults would be validated without compliance check, which would undermine the sanction set forth by the Paediatric Regulation. Therefore the Commission imposes partial compliance checks, that is, compliance with the PIP is checked each time a regulatory application is submitted, which is subject to Article 7 or 8 of the Paediatric Regulation.

In case of a PIP that covers more than one condition, the partial compliance check does not cover all the conditions but is limited to the condition of which the indication applied for is part. This practice has been strengthened by the EMA's Policy on the Scope of PIP decisions that requires matching the scope of the PIP and the scope of the regulatory application. In a nutshell, the company must request a modification of the PIP so that it is split into two PIPs: one PIP that covers the condition for which the regulatory application is submitted and one PIP with the other condition(s). The compliance check only concerns the first PIP. If that PIP is completed, the company is eligible for a reward.

4.2.4.3 Amendment to the SmPC (Art. 28(1) and 36(1))

This requirement means that the results of all the paediatric studies must be disclosed in the SmPC of the medicinal product. If the medicinal product is new and the PIP is completed before the submission of the MAA, the information will be in the initial SmPC. In all other cases, the initial SmPC will have to be amended.

In practice, this requirement is redundant with the requirement to have a compliance statement in the MA (see the preceding) since the amendment of the SmPC is a prerequisite for the inclusion of the compliance statement in the MA. We, therefore, will not provide lengthy explanations thereon. One point is worthwhile noting: the so-called procedure Article 29.

Article 29 of the Paediatric Regulation aims at speeding up the approval of the paediatric medicinal product in all the member states. Amending the SmPC is not so much an issue in cases of medicinal products authorised through the centralised procedure. It is much more burdensome in cases of medicinal products authorised through the decentralised procedure because each national MA must be amended and Article 36(1) requires that the paediatric product be authorised in all the member states. The procedure for amending the SmPC can be a line extension, a type II variation or another type of variation, depending on the change to be brought in the SmPC.

Applications for line extensions or type II variations to national MA must normally go through a decentralised procedure as well. However, changes linked to a PIP need not to follow the entire decentralised procedure—if the company wishes, the procedure may be limited to the arbitration by the CHMP. In such a case, the company files an application for variation or line extension with the EMA; the CHMP issues an opinion; the Commission takes a decision; and within 30 days, the member states must formally take a decision that is consistent with the Commission decision. The timetable is the same as for referrals under Article 30 of Directive 2001/83, but in practice, the procedure takes a minimum of 6 months.

4.2.4.4 Completion of significant studies after 26 January 2007 (Art. 45(3))

This requirement was temporary and became obsolete.

4.2.4.5 No orphan designation (Art. 36(4))

An orphan designation prevents an SPC extension. The Paediatric Regulation does not give the MAH of an orphan medicinal product that is patent protected, the choice of the reward: pursuant to Article 37, if the medicinal product has an orphan designation at the time of filing of the MAA, the reward is a market exclusivity extension. This situation, which is not that unusual, raises a few questions—see the succeeding text.

4.2.4.6 No '+1 year marketing protection' (Art. 36(5))

Medicinal products containing a new active substance are protected by 8 years of data exclusivity followed by 2 years of marketing protection. If a new indication that is considered to bring a significant benefit over the existing treatments is approved during the first 8 years of protection, the medicinal product benefits from an extra year of marketing protection (+1 year).

If that new indication is a paediatric indication developed on the basis of an agreed PIP, the MAH could, in principle, claim both the +1 year and the paediatric reward and thus be rewarded twice for conducting the same studies. In order to prevent such a double reward, the Paediatric Regulation specifies that "if the applicant applies for, and obtains, a one-year extension of the period of marketing protection for the medicinal product concerned, on the grounds that this new paediatric indication brings a significant clinical benefit in comparison with existing therapies, in accordance with Article 14(11) of Regulation (EC) No 726/2004 or the fourth subparagraph of Article 10(1) of Directive 2001/83/EC." The company may not rely on the same studies to claim both the +1 year of marketing protection and the SPC extension. It has to choose between one of those incentives, and if it opts for and obtains the +1 year, it is no longer eligible for the SPC extension.

The wording of Article 36(5) refers to a new paediatric indication and thus is clear that the prohibition is limited to cases where the +1 year of marketing protection is granted on the basis of the paediatric data generated by implementing a PIP. This reading is supported by the legislative history of the Paediatric Regulation.

Therefore, in theory, a company is not prevented from benefiting successively from the +1 year of data exclusivity and then from the SPC extension if it develops a new indication with a significant benefit and then a new paediatric indication. Furthermore, in the case of a full product development, the adult studies could be used to claim the +1 year, and the paediatric studies could be used to claim the SPC extension. Similarly, in the case of two different paediatric developments, albeit on the basis of the same

PIP, the paediatric studies for condition A could be used to claim the +1 year, and the paediatric studies for condition B could be used to claim the SPC extension.

The prohibition to claim both the +1 year and the paediatric reward is not included in Article 37 of the Paediatric Regulation; hence, strictly speaking, it should not apply if the reward is the market exclusivity extension.

Article 36(5) prohibits a double reward but does not specify when and how the company should choose between the SPC extension and the +1 year. On the other hand, the Commission has adopted a guideline on the +1-year pursuant to which a company wanting to obtain this additional protection must include in its regulatory application additional data proving that the new indication brings a significant therapeutic benefit.[k] Therefore, in practice, the company opts for the +1 year when submitting the regulatory application for the new indication. At that time, the company has no certainty that the SPC extension will be granted. If it opts for the SPC extension and does not submit the additional data and the SPC extension is later denied by the NPOs, the company can no longer claim the +1 year and thus is not rewarded for its paediatric development. Clearly, this system is not efficient and should be improved.

4.2.4.7 No previous SPC extension (Art. 52(9))

The Paediatric Reward only provides for one SPC extension per SPC.

4.2.4.8 Two-year time limit for the filing of the application for SPC extension

Article 52 of the Paediatric Regulation amended Article 7 of the SPC Regulation, which relates to the times at which applications for SPC extension can be filed.

The application for an SPC extension must be filed at least 2 years before the expiration of an SPC.

We note that for a transitional period of 5 years starting on 26 January 2007, the time limit was 6 months rather than 2 years. The objective of the transitional period was to allow existing products of the SPC, which were close to expiration to benefit from the paediatric reward as well. A similar transitional period now exists for Iceland and Norway.

4.2.4.9 Content of the application for SPC extension

Article 52 of the Paediatric Regulation amended Article 8.1 of the SPC Regulation by adding a new paragraph (d), which states that:

> where the application for a certificate includes a request for an extension of the duration:
> (i) a copy of the statement indicating compliance with an agreed completed paediatric investigation plan as referred to in Article 36(1) of Regulation (EC) No 1901/2006;

---

[k] European Commission, Guidance on elements required to support the significant clinical benefit in comparison with existing therapies of a new therapeutic indication in order to benefit from an extended (11 year) marketing protection period, Nov. 2007.

(ii) where necessary, in addition to the copy of the authorisations to place the product on the market as referred to in point (b), proof that it has authorisations to place the product on the market of all other Member States, as referred to in Article 36(3) of Regulation (EC) No 1901/2006.

As explained above, the SPC rules emanate from the EU but are implemented and interpreted at the national level. Thus it is for the NPOs to determine the meaning of Article 8(1)(d) and the documents with which they want to be provided for granting an SPC extension.

According to the Commission, the NPOs should require that the applicant submit (i) a MA that contains a compliance statement and (ii) proof that the paediatric product is approved in all the member states. The Commission also considers that those documents must be provided at the time of filing of the application for an SPC extension. Yet, national practices vary with regard to the documents that must be provided to prove that the compliance and approval requirements have been met (for instance, certain NPOs request copies of all the national MAs with translation into the local language while others accept self-certification). National practices also vary as to the point at which the documents must be provided (certain NPOs request the documents in the application for SPC extension, while others ask for them later on but within a specified time limit or even before the expiry of the SPC pursuant to Article 10(3) and (4) of the SPC Regulation).

Another important issue is whether the NPOs should check the fulfilment of the requirements set out by Article 36 (no orphan designation and no +1 year).

4.2.5 Market exclusivity extension: Substantive and procedural requirements

The general substantive requirements are the same as for the SPC extension.

No specific substantive requirement is set forth by Article 37 of the Paediatric Regulation. However, the EMA considers that the prohibition to benefit from both the +1 year and the SPC extension applies by analogy to the marketing exclusivity extension. Such an application by analogy is not acceptable because the European legislature has decided to mirror certain but not all requirements for SPC extensions, including the prohibition of the +1 year.

No procedural requirement applies either. The Paediatric Regulation does not foresee a specific procedure for claiming the +2 years of market exclusivity. The only procedural' requirement is that the market exclusivity has not expired.

4.2.6 PUMA (Art. 30 and 31)

For MAHs of approved/off-patent medicinal products that decided voluntarily to comply with the paediatric obligation and to complete a PIP, the Paediatric Regulation creates a new category of MAs, the PUMA (see the preceding text).

The PUMA application can be a hybrid application (abridged application with own paediatric data) or a mixed application (bibliographic application with own paediatric data). It can go through the centralised procedure. If the company has also developed other, nonpaediatric, indications, it may file another regulatory application for those indications but not through the centralised procedure.

One advantage of a PUMA is that the paediatric product may have the same brand name as the adult product (provided, of course, that the MAH is the same). The MAH of a well-known medicinal product for adults thus can benefit from having invested in marketing its adult product. Another advantage is that the PUMA is a specific MA, which is not covered by the global MA, which means that the new paediatric data are protected by 8 + 2 + 1 years (see the preceding text).

However, overall, it is commonly agreed that a PUMA is not an attractive reward. There are various reasons: off-label use of the adult version of the generic, difficulties in obtaining a satisfactory price and reimbursement, and competition from hospital preparations and the like. This explains the low number of PIPs for PUMAs and of granted PUMAs.

In addition, the PUMA raises a few questions. First, the EMA accepts that the PIP does not have to cover all the subsets of the paediatric population. In such a case, is the PUMA limited to the subsets of the paediatric population covered by the PIP? Second, the Commission considers that a PUMA precludes an orphan designation and *viceversa*. One may wonder about the legal provisions of the Paediatric Regulation or the Orphan Regulation on which this prohibition is based.

4.2.7 Main issues with the SPC extension

The application of the provisions on paediatric rewards raises many issues, some of which have already been examined previously. Other noteworthy issues are the following:

4.2.7.1 SPC with negative term

Article 13 of the SPC Regulation sets out the rule for calculating the term of SPCs and caps that term at 5 years as from the date of expiration of the patent. In practice, where an NPO receives an application for an SPC, it calculates the term of the SPC, and if the calculation does not lead to a positive result, it either informs the applicant and asks him to withdraw the application or declares that the application is invalid. This approach was recommended by the Commission in 1995 because a '0 term' SPC 'serves no useful purpose'.

Before the adoption of the Paediatric Regulation, this practice did not draw any attention. Companies were not interested in SPCs without a positive term because such an SPC was deemed to be worthless, while fees still had to be paid for obtaining and maintaining the SPC. The Paediatric Regulation changed the perspective because a '0 term' SPC could now be extended by 6 months.

In October 2006 and September 2008, the Commission stressed to the NPO that '0 term' SPCs should not be granted because an SPC had first to exist to be extended. Nevertheless, the discussion continued and was extended to the term of the SPC: should the term be zero or negative.

In 2011, the European Court of Justice disagreed with the Commission and ruled that NPOs may grant SPC with a negative term of a maximum 6 months in order to enable the SPC extension.[1]

4.2.7.2 Multiple SPCs

Normally, one SPC only may be granted per active ingredient or combination of active substances. However, in practice, several SPCs are sometimes delivered for a same active substance, to different patent holders. Insofar as the same active substance can be protected by several SPCs, logically an SPC extension can be applied for by each SPC holder. This is confirmed by the Commission (see Minutes NPO Meeting).

4.2.7.3 Convergence between the scope of the SPC and the scope of the MA

Another question is whether an extension of the SPC can be based on an MA covering a condition or a therapeutic indication that is different from the condition or therapeutic indication covered by the PIP. The answer should be yes, as the Paediatric Regulation does not contain such a restriction. Along the same lines, is the scope of protection afforded by the SPC extension the same as that of the SPC or only the paediatric formulation covered by the PIP? The Danish Maritime and Commercial Court has considered that the SPC extension has the same scope of protection as the SPC it extends, rightfully so, as the SPC extension is simply meant to prolong the term of the SPC by 6 months.

4.2.8 Main issues with the market exclusivity extension

Orphan products raise several issues, especially with regard to paediatric reward. Orphan medicinal products are the poor relatives of the Paediatric Regulation. Not only is the implementation of a PIP especially burdensome for an orphan company, but also the reward is somewhat uncertain and raises many questions.

4.2.8.1 New indication of an authorised orphan medicinal product

The Paediatric Regulation does not expressly provide for a reward in the case of a new indication of an authorised orphan medicinal product: Article 37 of the Paediatric Regulation seems limited to new orphan products, and Article 8 applies to medicinal products that are SPC or patent protected. This clearly is an oversight because the Paediatric Regulation obviously has to incentivise the development of new indications, formulations, or routes of administration of approved orphan products.

At first, the Commission considered that new indication of authorised orphan medicinal products could not benefit from a market exclusivity extension if the medicinal

---

[1] ECJ, 8 Dec. 2011, *MSD*, C-215/10.

product was not protected by an SPC or a patent that qualified for an SPC.[m] However, the Commission changed its mind and now considers that a market exclusivity extension rather than a PUMA may be granted.

4.2.8.2 Reward for a patented orphan medicinal product

A different reward was established for orphan medicinal products on the assumption that those products are not usually protected by patents and, therefore, may not obtain SPC extensions (see Recital 29). Yet, some orphan medicinal products are patent protected. When a medicinal product is protected by an SPC or a patent that qualifies for an SPC and has an orphan designation, one would expect that the company is able to choose their paediatric reward. This is not the case.

Article 37 states that "[w]here an application for MA is submitted in respect of a medicinal product designated as an orphan medicinal product pursuant to Regulation (EC) No 141/200," the reward is +2 years of market exclusivity, and Article 36(4) of the Paediatric Regulation prevents the SPC extension if the medicinal product has an orphan designation. The MAH of an orphan product that is SPC or patent protected, therefore, does not choose the reward: if the medicinal product has an orphan designation when the MAA is filed, the reward is +2 years of market exclusivity.

An SPC, however, covers the active ingredient and so protects all the medicinal products that contain that ingredient, while the market exclusivity extension only covers the medicinal product with the orphan designation. An SPC extension, therefore, is usually more valuable than a market exclusivity extension (subject to other considerations such as pricing and reimbursement). In such a case, the only option for the company is to remove voluntarily the orphan designation before filing the MAA for the (previously orphan) medicinal product. Such a voluntary removal is expressly permitted by Article 5(12) of the Orphan Regulation.

The voluntary withdrawal of the orphan designation raises a couple of issues. First, a medicinal product may have been granted several orphan designations. Should all the orphan designations be removed? The answer should be no, as the PIP covers one rare condition and only the market exclusivity relating to that condition will benefit from the market exclusivity extension. Second, several regulatory submissions are generally submitted before a PIP is completed. At what point should the orphan designation be removed? To the extent that Article 37 refers to an MAA containing the results of all the measures contained in the PIP, the orphan designation should be removed up until (i.e., right before) the last regulatory submission under the PIP. Third, can the company benefit from the SPC extension if it has removed the orphan designation but benefited from market exclusivity, be it partly (less than 10 years) or partly? That question was answered positively by the Interim Judge of the District Court of The Hague on 30 March 2016 in the case of *Novartis* v *Teva*.[n]

We note that the Commission found a compromise to avoid systematic withdrawals of orphan designations and proposed another solution for medicinal products with

---

[m] GC, 3 Sept. 2014, *Shire*, T-583/13.
[n] District Court of the Hague, 30 March 2016, *Novartis AG v Teva BV et al.*

patent protection and an orphan designation, that is, file two PIPs, one for orphan indications whose completion triggers an ME extension and one for nonorphan indications whose completion triggers an SPC extension. This solution mirrors the requirement set forth in the Orphan Regulation to have a MA for orphan indications and another MA for nonorphan indications.[o] We will not comment at length on that solution. We however point out that, under such a solution, the 'Orphan PIP' submitted for a new orphan indication of an authorised product must be based on Article 7 so that the paediatric obligation applies, even if the product is already authorised and is no longer patent protected.

4.2.8.3 Reduction of market exclusivity

What is the interaction between the 2-year market exclusivity extension and the reduction of the market exclusivity from 10 to 6 years? The market exclusivity may be reduced to 6 years if, 'at the end of the fifth year, it is established, in respect of the medicinal product concerned, that the designation criteria laid down in Article 3 are no longer met, *inter alia*, where it is shown on the basis of available evidence that the product is sufficiently profitable not to justify maintenance of market exclusivity' (Article 8(2) of the Orphan Regulation).

According to the Commission, the additional years of market exclusivity for paediatric development are added to the 10-year period, and the reduction applies to that period so that the reduction foreseen in Article 8(2) of the Orphan Regulation leads to 6 and not 8 years of market exclusivity. In other words, the reduction of market exclusivity will also annihilate the market exclusivity extension. However, even under this interpretation, the MAH could arguably benefit from 8 years of market exclusivity if the reduction to 6 years occurs before the paediatric development.

4.2.9 More than one paediatric reward?

A final interesting issue is whether a company may benefit from more than one paediatric reward. The Paediatric Regulation expressly prevents more than one SPC extension per SPC, but it does not prevent, even implicitly, a company from being granted successive paediatric rewards.

Obviously, this should only be possible if the company completes more than one PIP. For instance, a company would benefit from an SPC extension if it completed a PIP for, say, the treatment of headache in children and, after expiry of the SPC extension, developed the active substance for the treatment of cystic fibrosis and benefited from a market exclusivity extension further to completion of a PIP for treatment of cystic fibrosis. The Commission or the EMA would probably try opposing such successive rewards even though they alone incentivise paediatric research beyond the first paediatric indication.

---

[o] Pursuant to Article 7(3) of the Orphan Regulation No. 141/2000, a same MA may not include orphan and nonorphan indications.

4.3 Are the paediatric rewards adapted?

The Paediatric Regulation was meant to balance obligations and rewards so that companies would be compensated for their mandatory investment in paediatric development and incentivised to invest in optional paediatric development. One can safely say that things did not go according to plan because the rewards are not well adapted to their objectives and are too hard to obtain.

The inadequacy of the paediatric rewards is multifaced, for example:

- The Report on 10 Years of Application of the Paediatric Regulation published by the Commission in October 2017[p] concludes on an average investment of about 20 million euros per PIP, which is five times more than initially calculated and relied upon for determining the duration of the SPC extension. The only conclusion is that the term of the SPC extension is not long enough to compensate the investment.
- The same Commission's report acknowledges that the PUMA is a failure. This clearly results from the very low number of PIP for PUMA and even lower number of PUMA granted so far (seven). This is a very important issue because most of the medicinal products on the market today still are approved/off-patent medicinal products.
- The Paediatric Regulation does not provide a reward for new medicinal products that have neither patent protection nor orphan designation. The most striking example is vaccines, which, in addition, are typically paediatric medicinal products.
- The market exclusivity extension may be an adequate reward for orphan medicinal products, but completing PIPs for orphan medicinal products is very challenging and may result in the market exclusivity having expired before completion of the PIP.

A better analysis of the adequacy of the paediatric rewards will be possible after the Commission publishes the results of its study on the combined effects of the Paediatric Regulation and the Orphan Regulation and its study on the Orphan Regulation. It is hoped that the Commission will fix the issues.

We also note that since the entry into force of the Paediatric Regulation in 2007, more than 1500 PIPs have been agreed by the EMA, while only about 70 rewards have been granted,[q] many of them recently. The reasons for such striking unbalance are complex. An obvious cause is the stringent legal requirements for being eligible for a reward, which, in addition, are interpreted restrictively by the Commission. Another cause is long deferrals. According to the Commission and the EMA, paediatric rewards only start being granted now, after several years of application of the Paediatric Regulation because PIPs first had to be completed and long deferrals has been accepted. However, the need for long deferrals was (and is) due to the EMA being very demanding with regard to the nature, the number, and the features (number of patients, endpoints, etc.) of the paediatric studies and very restrictive with regard to waivers. Had the EMA been less demanding, many more PIPs would have been completed by now. To date, many PIPs are still ongoing that hopefully will soon trigger paediatric rewards, and restore, albeit slightly, the unbalance between PIPs and paediatric rewards.

---

[p] See footnote d.
[q] At the end of 2017, about 50 SPC extensions, 7 market exclusivity extensions, and 7 PUMAs had been granted.

While the delay in obtaining the rewards does not directly concern the adequacy of the rewards, it illustrates another drawback of the system set up by the Paediatric Regulation.

4.4 Switzerland

4.4.1 Introduction

Switzerland is a member of the major patent-related international treaties and conventions. This includes, for example, the Paris Convention for the Protection of Industrial Property, the Agreement on the Trade-Related Aspects of Intellectual Property Rights, the Patent Cooperation Treaty, or the European Patent Convention (EPC). Together with Liechtenstein, Switzerland forms a unified territory for patent protection.[r] A national or a European patent according to the EPC "may only be granted, transferred, annulled, or lapse in respect of the whole territory of protection."[s]

Switzerland is not part of the EU, nor of the European Economic Area (EEA). Switzerland's relation to the EU is based on bilateral sectoral agreements. Generally the agreements related to market access are governed by existing EU law, and Switzerland has undertaken to enact equivalent provisions or to adopt existing EU law. Outside this framework, the country pursues a policy of autonomous adoption of EU law where appropriate. For example, in 1995, Switzerland adopted the substantive content of Regulation No. 1768/92 concerning the supplementary protection certificate for medicinal products (now Regulation No. 469/2009).[t]

Ten years after the EU, in 2016, Switzerland adopted its incentive system for paediatric medicinal products. It required changes in the Swiss Patens Act (PatA)[u] and the Swiss Therapeutic Products Act (TPA).[v] Based on the understanding that in Switzerland, children should also have access to medicinal products that are specifically tailored to their needs and the Swiss legislator introduced several measures to encourage innovation that leads to new paediatric treatments, rather than off-label uses of adult medicines. The introduced changes in the PatA and the TPA aim to encourage and reward the development of medicinal products for the paediatric population and to improve access to the information related to the use of such products for children. The paediatric extensions reward pharmaceutical producers for conducting paediatric studies according to an approved PIP.

---

[r] Treaty between the Swiss Confederation and the Principality of Liechtenstein on Patent Protection (Patent Treaty) from December 22, 1978, at https://www.wipo.int/edocs/lexdocs/treaties/en/ch-li/trt_ch_li.pdf.
[s] Art. 4 of the treaty between the Swiss Confederation and the Principality of Liechtenstein on Patent Protection (Patent Treaty) from December 22, 1978.
[t] Council Regulation (EEC) No. 1768/92 of 18 June 1992 concerning the creation of a supplementary protection certificate for medicinal products, now Regulation (EC) of the European Parliament and of the Council of 6 May 2009 concerning the supplementary protection certificate for medicinal products.
[u] Federal Act on Patents for Inventions (Patents Act, PatA), SR 232.14, at https://www.admin.ch/opc/en/classified-compilation/19540108/index.html.
[v] Federal Act on Medicinal Products and Medical Devices (Therapeutic Products Act, TPA), SR 812.21, at https://www.admin.ch/opc/en/classified-compilation/20002716/index.html.

The revised TPA introduced the necessary additional requirements for MA in Switzerland, amongst others, the obligation to perform paediatric studies based on an agreed PIP (Art. 54a TPA).

Both the revised PatA and TPA entered into force on 1 January 2019, together with the related Patent Ordinance[w] and the guidelines for the substantive examination of national patent applications[x] of the Swiss Federal Institute of Intellectual Property.

4.4.2 Regulatory framework

The revision of the TPA introduced the obligation to develop and submit a PIP and to carry out studies for paediatric use (Art. 54a TPA). The Swiss system is implemented on the basis of EU Regulation (EC) No. 1901/2006. Applicants have two options: they can either submit a PIP that has already been approved by a foreign medicines agency with comparable medicinal product control, or they can develop their own PIP. PIPs approved by a foreign medicines agency with comparable medicinal product control are accepted by the Swiss Agency for Therapeutic Products (Swissmedic) without a separate review.

The obligation to submit a PIP applies to the following applications (Art. 5 para. 2 Ordinance on the Therapeutic Products,[y] hereinafter TPO):

- for MA of a medicinal product containing at least one new active substance in the ordinary procedure;
- for MA of an important orphan medicinal product containing at least one new active substance;
- for authorisation of a new indication, a new pharmaceutical form or a new route of administration of a medicinal product as referred to in points previously mentioned.

As mentioned, this obligation is also fulfilled if the applicant submits a PIP approved by a country or agency designated by Swissmedic with comparable medicinal product control (Art. 5 para. 3 TPO). Accepted agencies are, for example, the European Medicines Agency or the Food and Drug Agency.

Swissmedic can grant a specific waiver of the obligation to produce a PIP or carry out studies for individual paediatric indications or development stages (partial waiver) in certain cases, for example, when the disease to be treated by the medicinal product only occurs in adults, when there is evidence that the medicinal product is likely to be ineffective in the paediatric population or its use appears questionable for safety reasons, or when the medicinal product is not expected to offer any significant therapeutic benefit over existing paediatric treatments.

---

[w] Only available in German, French, Italian; in German: Verordnung über die Erfindungspatente, SR 232.141, at https://www.admin.ch/opc/de/classified-compilation/19770250/index.html; also in French or Italian.

[x] Only available in German or French; in German: Richtlinien für die Sachprüfung nationalen Patentanmeldungen, at https://www.ige.ch/fileadmin/user_upload/schuetzen/patente/d/richtlinien_patente/RiLi_Sachpruefung_CH-Patent_DE_201901.pdf.

[y] Only in German, French, Italian; in German: Verordnung über die Arzneimittel (Arzneimittelverordnung, VAM), SR 812.212.21, at https://www.admin.ch/opc/de/classified-compilation/20173471/index.html.

It is also possible to request a deferral of the initiation or completion of some or all of the measures set out in the PIP. The aim is to ensure that studies are conducted only if they are safe and ethically acceptable and that the (planned) paediatric studies do not delay the MA of medicinal products for other population groups. The deferrals are granted on request. An applicant is required to provide appropriate justification, such as ensuring public health, and scientific or technical arguments are considered as possible grounds, for deferral.[z]

The applicant is obliged to continually update the relevant positive or negative results from studies conducted in accordance with the approved PIP in suitable form in the information for healthcare professionals, (Art. 28 TPO).

4.4.3 Types of paediatric rewards

For the background on the SPC and data exclusivity, I refer to the explanations provided in Chapter B. (1).

4.4.3.1 SPC and paediatric extensions

As previously mentioned, Switzerland autonomously adopted the substantive EU legislation on SPC. The requirements for the grant of a Swiss SPC correspond to those according to Regulation (EC) No. 469/2009. With the revision of the PatA in 2016, the Swiss legislator intended to introduce the EU system of paediatric extension. The initial draught of the new legislation referred to the extension of a SPC for 6 month if paediatric studies have been performed. During the Parliamentary discussions, a new form of protection was introduced, the so-called paediatric SPC. This new SPC aims to incentivise R&D for paediatric indications and to provide a reward for the performed paediatric studies according to the PIP in cases where no regular SPC exists. The Swiss legislator intended to avoid the complexity of negative term SPC[aa] and their extensions and considered that the full 6-month protection should apply when paediatric studies have been performed.

The established paediatric extension system in Switzerland provides now two options:

- a paediatric extension of a SPC for 6 months;
- an independent paediatric SPC, which is directly linked to the basic patent when no regular SPC exists also valid for 6 months.

4.4.3.2 Data exclusivity for exclusively paediatric medicinal products

Switzerland provides data exclusivity for a medicinal product containing at least one new active substance for 10 years (Art. 11a TPA). There are different protection terms in special cases, such as exclusively paediatric products or medicinal products for rare

---

[z] For further information see Swissmedic Guidance document Paediatric investigation plan HMV4, at https://www.swissmedic.ch/dam/swissmedic/en/dokumente/zulassung/zl_hmv_iv/zl000_00_023d_wlpaediatirschespruefkonzept.pdf.download.pdf/zl000_00_023e_wlpaediatricinvestigationplan.pdf.
[aa] CJEU C-125/10 Merck Sharp & Dohme Corporation, 8 December 2011.

diseases (Art. 11b TPA). Pursuant to Art. 11b para. 1 TPA and Art. 30 para. 2 TPO, a protection period of 3 years is granted for extensions of approval or amendments including new indication, new route of administration, new dosage form, new dose strength, or new recommended dosage. With respect to paediatric medicinal products, Switzerland allows simultaneous use, contrary to the EU, of both forms of protection, that is, a paediatric extension and data exclusivity for medicinal products that are exclusively for paediatric use (Art. 11b para. 3 TPA).

4.4.3.3 Orphan medicinal products

A disease is considered rare in Switzerland if occurs in less than 5 cases per 10,000 inhabitants and is life-threatening or chronically debilitating. Switzerland system on incentivizing product development for rare diseases includes data exclusivity, waiver of fees for their authorisation (Art. 65 para. 5 TPA, Art. 9 lit. a of the Ordinance on Therapeutic Products Fees[ab]), and the possibility of obtaining scientific support from Swissmedic (Art. 25 of the ordinance on the simplified authorisation of medicinal products and the authorisation of medicinal products in the notification procedure). It does not provide market exclusivity as in the EU.

Art. 14 para. 1 lit. f TPA states that important medicinal products for rare diseases are eligible for the simplified authorisation procedure. The recognition of the status as an important medicinal product for rare diseases is regulated in Articles 4–7 TPLO[ac] and the authorisation of a related medicinal product in Articles 24–26 TPLO.[ad]

4.4.4 Swiss paediatric extensions system: Substantive and procedural requirements

4.4.4.1 Paediatric extension of a SPC

The new Articles 140n–140s of the revised PatA are partly inspired by the EU Paediatric Drug Regulation (EC) No. 1901/2006.[ae] The grant of a **paediatric extension of a SPC** is subject to the following requirements:

- A basic patent in force, a Swiss MA with the corresponding PIP, and a SPC;
- The applicant must provide a confirmation issued by Swissmedic that the product information contains the results of the studies performed according to the paediatric investigation plan (new Art. 140n para. 1 lit. a).

[ab] Updated version not yet available in English; in German: Verordnung des Schweizerischen Heilmittelinstituts über seine Gebühren (GebV-Swissmedic), SR 812.214.5, at https://www.admin.ch/opc/de/classified-compilation/20173463/201901010000/812.214.5.pdf.

[ac] Ordinance of the Swiss Agency for Therapeutic Products of 22 June 2006 on the Simplified Licensing of Therapeutic Products and the Licensing of Therapeutic Products by the Notification Procedure, SR 812.212.23.

[ad] For further information see Swissmedic document "Guidance document Orphan Drug HMV4", at https://www.swissmedic.ch/dam/swissmedic/en/dokumente/zulassung/zl_hmv_iv/zl100_00_002d_wleorphan-drugs.pdf.download.pdf/ZL100_00_002e_WL%20Guidance%20document%20Orphan%20Drug.pdf.

[ae] Regulation (EC) No. 1901/2006 of the European Parliament and of the Council on medicinal products for paediatric use, 12 December 2006.

Swissmedic provides the written confirmation on request if all the conditions set out in the PIP are fulfilled and the knowledge obtained on paediatric use is fully incorporated in the information for healthcare professionals in the appropriate form (Art. 9 para. 5 TPO). The applicant must provide a summary table of fulfilment of the conditions after the last PIP condition has been fulfilled, including all measures listed in the PIP; the abbreviated results of studies; the Swissmedic official decision (date and application ID) on the fulfilment of the measures; and a list of changes, in keywords, in the information for healthcare professionals and patient information, including mention of negative study results.[af]
- The Swiss MA application must be filed within 6 months after the application for a relevant MA in the EEA (Art. 140n para. 1 lit. b). This provision is a particularity of the Swiss law that intends to speed up access to new drugs for children. An applicant will have to provide documentation including the information on the filing date in the EEA, on the active ingredient and the related PIP (Chapter 13.2.5 Guidelines for the Substantive Examination of National Patent Applications, hereafter Guidelines). There are three exceptions to this link between the MA application in the EEA and the one in Switzerland (Chapter 13.2.5 Guidelines): (1) No EEA MA application has been filed prior to the Swiss MA application; (2) the Swiss MA with the corresponding PIP has been filed within 6 months after the entry into force of the revised PatA (deadline is June 30, 2019); in this case, the temporal connection with an EEA MA application is no taken into account (transitional provision Art. 149 para. 3); (3) the MA application with the corresponding PIP has been submitted to Swissmedic prior to the entry into force of the revised PatA. In this case, the application is deemed to have been filed on the day of the entry into force. Art. 149 para. 3 PatA is applied, that is, the 6-month period between the EEA application and the Swiss application is not considered.
- The paediatric extension of a SPC can be filed together with the application for the underlying SPC or at the latest 2 years before the expiry of the SPC (Art. 140 o para. 1). During a transition period of 5 years after the entry into force of the new legislation, the time limit for an application is 6 months before the SPC expiry date (Art. 149 para. 1).

4.4.4.2 Paediatric SPC

Deviating from the EU system of paediatric extension, Switzerland introduced, in addition to the paediatric extension of a SPC, an independent **paediatric supplementary protection certificate (P-SPC)**.

The P-SPC is directly linked to the basic patent and starts upon patent expiry. It can be obtained if no ordinary SPC has been granted for the same product (Art. 140v para. 3, Art. 140a para. 1). The legal effect of the P-SPC is the same as of a regular SPC, that is, it is not limited to the paediatric use. The P-SPC is granted for 6 months.

The grant requirements for a P-SPC are largely identical to those of a regular SPC and the paediatric extension of a SPC:

- A basic patent in force; a Swiss MA (not necessarily the first one).
- The applicant must provide the confirmation of Swissmedic that the product information contains the results of all tests performed based on the PIP (see Section 4.4.4.1).

[af] For further information see Swissmedic Guidance document Paediatric investigation plan HMV4, at https://www.swissmedic.ch/dam/swissmedic/en/dokumente/zulassung/zl_hmv_iv/zl000_00_023d_wlpaediatirschespruefkonzept.pdf.download.pdf/zl000_00_023e_wlpaediatricinvestigationplan.pdf.

- Respecting the deadline of 6 months between the filing of the EEA MA application with PIP and the relevant Swiss MA application (see Section 4.4.4.1);
- In addition, the P-SPC is subject to the substantive requirements of an ordinary SPC (Art. 140v para. 3, Art. 140b para. 1), that is, in particular the product must be protected by a basic patent.
- If the patent proprietor is not the MA holder (recipient of the Swissmedic certification under Art. 140t para. 1), he must provide a letter of consent of the MA holder regarding the P-SPC application (Art. 140u para. 3). This provision has been included to ensure that the reward of a paediatric extension goes to the party that has actually performed the paediatric studies.
- No regular SPC has been granted for the same active ingredient to the same patent holder (Art. 140a para. 1 second sentence). A regular SPC and a P-SPC are mutually exclusive.
- Time line for filing: The application for a P-SPC can be filed after the grant of the patent and the MA or at the latest 2 years before the expiry of the basic patent. During the transition period of 5 years, the time limit for filing is 6 months before patent expiry (Art. 149 para. 2).
- The transition rule in Art. 149 para. 3 also applies for P-SPCs, that is, the link between EEA MA application and the Swiss MA application will not be examined if the Swiss MA (or the PIP) has been filed within the first 6 months after entry into force of the revised PatA.

4.4.5 Swiss data exclusivity for paediatric medicinal products: Substantive and procedural requirements

As previously mentioned, contrary to the EU, Switzerland does not exclude data exclusivity if a paediatric extension has been granted. The TPA provides data exclusivity for 10 years for medicinal products that are exclusively for paediatric use, provided no data exclusivity has been granted for another medicine with the same active pharmaceutical ingredient and the same special paediatric application (Art. 11b para. 3 TPA, Art. 30 TPO). Data exclusivity is granted regardless of whether the paediatric medicinal product contains a new or known active ingredient.

The prerequisite for the grant is that the submitted studies comply with the agreed PIP and that all measures according to the PIP have been fulfilled.

Data exclusivity is only possible for exclusively paediatric medicinal products for which the MA application has been submitted after the entry into force of the revised TPA in January 2019 (Art. 86 TPO).

The application for data exclusivity can be submitted as part of the MA application. It is possible to apply for data exclusivity for paediatric medicinal products that have already received a MA. In this case the calculation of the 10 years protection term will be based on the date of the MA decision of the paediatric medicine.[ag]

Swissmedic publishes the type and the duration of the data exclusivity for an exclusively paediatric medicinal product on its webpage.

In case a MA holder intends to discontinue the marketing of an exclusively paediatric medicinal product for which data exclusivity protection has been granted, this intention must be published in an appropriate form (Art. 16a para. 4 TPA). In addition,

---

[ag] For further information see Swissmedic document "Wegleitung Unterlagenschutz HMV4", currently in German only, at https://www.swissmedic.ch/dam/swissmedic/de/dokumente/zulassung/zl_hmv_iv/zl000_00_024d_wlunterlagenschutz.pdf.download.pdf/zl000_00_024d_wlunterlagenschutz.pdf.

it must be publicly announced that the relevant documentation will be made available to third parties free of charge for the purpose of obtaining their own marketing authorisation (Art. 16a para. 5 TPA). This legal provision aims to ensure that paediatric medicinal products remain available in Switzerland even after the expiry of the data exclusivity protection and/or SPC, including paediatric extensions granted to them.[ah]

4.4.6 Data exclusivity for an orphan medicinal products

The Swiss TPA provides data exclusivity of 15 years for important medicinal products for rare disease (Art. 11b para. 4 TPA), provided that no exclusivity protection has been granted to another approved product with the same active pharmaceutical ingredient and the same therapeutic application.

The data exclusivity application becomes part of the MA application if provided together. An exclusivity application can also be submitted after the MA of the medicinal product. However, the protection term calculation will be based on the date of the MA decision for the orphan medicinal product.

The data exclusivity regulation applies only to important orphan medicinal products that have been applied for after the entry into force of the revised TPA in January 2019 (Art. 86 Ordinance on Medicinal Products).

Swissmedic will publish the type and duration of the data protection for an important orphan medicinal product at its homepage.

4.4.7 Final remark

Switzerland's incentive system for paediatric medicinal product is fairly new. In this respect, it is not yet possible to assess its effectiveness and impact. The Swiss legislator introduced some new approaches, including the P-SPC or data exclusivity for exclusively paediatric drugs that can be provided in parallel to the rewards according to the patent law. In addition, the recognition of foreign PIPs will speed up the MA process. It remains to be seen if these measures will accomplish their purpose.

[ah] See Swissmedic document "Wegleitung Unterlagenschutz HMV4", currently in German only, at https://www.swissmedic.ch/dam/swissmedic/de/dokumente/zulassung/zl_hmv_iv/zl000_00_024d_wlunterlagenschutz.pdf.download.pdf/zl000_00_024d_wlunterlagenschutz.pdf.

Child and adolescent psychopharmacology at the beginning of the 21st century

Anna I Parachikova[a], Philippe Auby[b]
[a]UCB Nordic A/S, Neurology Business Unit, Copenhagen, Denmark, [b]Otsuka Pharmaceutical Development & Commercialisation Europe, Frankfurt am Main, Germany

5.1 Introduction

Mental health disorders account for 30% of the nonfatal disease burden worldwide (WHO, 2016) and importantly are not solely disorders of adulthood, but instead exhibit additionally high prevalence in child and adolescent life. Paediatric mental health disorders are estimated to afflict 10%–20% of youth worldwide (Kieling et al., 2011), thereby representing a substantial global burden. In addition to the high prevalence during youth, most paediatric disorders persist into adulthood (Costello et al., 2011). Mental health challenges in children and adolescents thus have long-term consequences for the individual, families, and society as a whole.

The burden of the paediatric mental disorders is often associated with a lifetime of comorbidities and vocational and social challenges. Early-onset mental health disorders impact cognitive, emotional, and behavioural trajectories. Thus a framework encompassing biological-psychological-social networks with a neurobiological underpinning is vital when considering optimal management in youth aimed at high quality of life.

Evidence today demonstrates that psychopharmacology initiated early in life as part of multidisciplinary management confers long-term secondary prevention by diminishing unfavourable developmental trajectories.

We consider attention deficit hyperactivity disorder (ADHD) probably the best paradigm to discuss child and adolescent psychopharmacology at the beginning of the 21st century as it perfectly reflects mental health challenges throughout the lifespan especially as pharmacological treatment has robustly demonstrated long-term benefits. ADHD is associated with high risk for deviant behaviours (Barkley et al., 2004), and evidence to date demonstrates that pharmacological treatment reduces criminality rates by up to 40% (Lichtenstein et al., 2012).

Bradley in 1937 reported on the beneficial effects of the stimulant Benzedrine on ADHD symptomatology: "Possibly the most striking change in behaviour during the week of Benzedrine therapy occurred in the school activities of many of these patients… The improvement was noted in all school subjects. It appeared promptly on the first day Benzedrine was given and disappeared on the first day it was discontinued" (Bradley, 1937). Importantly, Bradley's (1937) initial observation of the clinical response of stimulants still holds to date. Since then, however, innovative treatment has been limited, and ADHD patient management while improved with current mediation remains in need of a holistic approach to care encompassing biological-psychological-social networks.

In conclusion, in children and adolescents suffering from psychiatric disturbances, pharmacological treatment represents a vital component of a multidimensional management plan supporting improvement in the quality of life.

5.2 Historical and cultural perspective

The first hospital specialising in the paediatric population was established in 1802 in Paris (Rey et al., 2015). Since the time of the first paediatric hospital, rapid growth in research and innovation has marked the field of child and adolescent psychiatry (Naveed et al., 2017). Between 1980 and 2016 the most commonly cited psychopathologies were found to include but not be limited to ADHD, anxiety, depression, and bipolar disorder, and methylphenidate was identified as the top keyword in child psychiatry (Naveed et al., 2017). Over the years, there has been a rapid development in literature focused on neurobiology, neuroimaging, genetics, and assessment tools and etiology within psychiatry. This multidimensional trend and innovative approaches can pave the way to improved psychopharmacological management early in life leading to improved quality in life.

The serendipitous discovery of amphetamine effects in diminishing hyperactivity in children in 1937 by Bradley to the 2000s clinical trials, paediatric psychopharmacology has become an active area of clinical practice. Importantly, during the last decade, the prescription rate for psychotropic medication has dramatically increased (Olfson et al., 2014; Rani et al., 2008). Here, specifically ADHD medication has seen a primary surge. The surge in stimulants has however also been marked by the growing concerns among the public and clinicians focused on the appropriateness of using such medication during the development period for not only physical but also emotional well-being (Kociancic et al., 2004; Arango, 2015). In addition to concerns of using stimulants on the developing brain, a further area of focus is on the surge representing overprescription or perhaps even abuse of the medication. However, analysis of available data has concluded that there is little evidence of these claims and that instead underuse may be a more significant problem in part of the United States and Europe (Goldman et al., 1998; Jensen et al., 1999; Adesman, 2001; Ekman and Gustafsson, 2000; Llana and Crismon, 1999; Biederman et al., 2008; Wilens et al., 2008).

Youth pharmacotherapy usage for mental disorders is highly variable worldwide. The variability in usage is the result of multiple factors including not only prevalence but also cultural, economic, and contextual variability, which modulates the decision-making process (Vitiello, 2008). The use of psychotropic medication is notably higher in developed countries with the United States representing 80% of the worldwide usage of stimulant medication. In addition to stimulants, the United

States is marked by the highest use of both antipsychotic and antidepressant medication (Fegert et al., 2006). While one in four cases is attended to in developed countries, access in low income/developing countries has been found to be 20 times lower. Additionally, experience and expertise for the optimal management of children and adolescents are limited in developing countries, and thus only a fraction of patients receive pharmacological treatment (WHO, 1975). Finally, in 2011, Jensen and colleagues published an epidemiological study describing a child mental health gap in the United States (Jensen et al., 2011). In conclusion, mental health management in children and adolescents is heterogeneous throughout the globe mainly due to cultural factors, and this diversity has implications for disease management and prognosis.

5.3 Development of child and adolescent treatments

Children and adolescents with psychotic disorders generally require pharmacological treatment to control symptoms of the disease with the aim of restoring functioning and improving the quality of life. Today, available medication options to treat mental conditions are not curative, but few symptomatic agents are available for the treatment of paediatric psychiatric disorders (for review, please see Persico et al., 2015). In contrast to adulthood, pharmacological treatment options do however remain spare for children and adolescents.

With the notable exception of stimulant medication, psychotropic medications were first developed to treat depression, anxiety, and psychosis in adults, which have thereupon been used in children. Thus paediatric pharmacology to date has been driven by either (a) serendipitous discovery or (b) medication label extensions from approval in adult population into the child and adolescent period.

Stimulant medication as previously noted has been uniquely positioned as the serendipitous finding in children, which later broadened into adulthood. Stimulants do represent the first pharmacological treatment initiated in children. Since its discovery in 1937, stimulants have remained the gold standard for the treatment of ADHD throughout the lifespan and in clinical studies have been associated with a large effect size (Faraone and Glatt, 2010). In the last 80 years, many modifications have occurred focusing on the formulation to provide long-lasting and consistent efficacy of stimulants. Importantly, however, while stimulants have now been accepted to play a vital part in the treatment of ADHD, treatment does not result in full functional improvement (Sikirica et al., 2015; Gjervan et al., 2012). In contrast to ADHD drugs, psychotropics have not been initiated in the paediatric population. In general, medication which was identified as being safe and efficacious in adults was adapted to be used in paediatric indication. In the last decades, clinical research has generated a substantial amount of evidence for the efficacy of pharmacological agents in children and adolescents. Importantly, however, the evidence of long-term efficacy and safety is of primary importance in child and adolescent pharmacology since as noted mental diseases first observed in children more often than not persist into the adulthood.

5.4 Challenges in child and adolescent psychopharmacology

Developmental psychopharmacology has evolved from considering children as "small adults" to acknowledging and developing options explicitly tailored to youth. The childhood and adolescence period is marked by immense not only physical but also psychosocial growth.

Developmental processes exert influences on absorption, distribution, metabolism, and excretion of molecular entities. Therefore direct translation of adult dosage to children may result in inadequate treatment. In children the relative mass of liver and kidney is higher than in adults when adjusting for body weight. Furthermore a drug's volume of distribution is greater in children compared with adults because of the different body water, fat, and plasma albumin levels between the two populations. In general, children are marked by lower bioavailability, faster metabolism, and elimination. The faster elimination will modulate the half-time of compounds. In adolescence, we have the additional challenge of the redistribution of body compartments and the gender differences in total body water and fat levels.

Pharmacological treatment for mental illnesses in children and adolescents most often act via modulation of neurotransmitters, the receptors of which undergo significant changes during the developmental period (Rho and Storey, 2001). Neurotransmitter receptor density peaks in childhood and then declines throughout adolescence, which is suggestive of potentially differential efficacy and safety throughout the lifespan. An example here is the observed difference in tolerability and efficacy of methylphenidate for the treatment of ADHD in children aged 3–5 years compared with older youth (Greenhill et al., 2006).

Lastly, medication approval is based on well-designed controlled studies demonstrating efficacy in reducing symptoms associated with a mental disorder. Recovery and improved functioning, however, are based not solely on improved symptomatology. There are though few studies showing effectiveness in recovery for stimulants in ADHD (Swanson et al., 2001) and antidepressants in adolescent depression (Kennard et al., 2006; Vitiello et al., 2006). In addition to the need of demonstrated efficacy, safety is especially important in youth. Pharmacological treatment during a period of vast development changes may be linked to additional toxicity concerns compared with adults, and thus long-term safety is a primary part of child and adolescent psychopharmacology.

5.5 Unmet needs in child and adolescent pharmacology

In 2013 the European Child and Adolescent Neuropsychopharmacology Network initiated a targeted network meeting to identify treatment gaps which culminated in the publication of the article by Persico et al. (2015). This highly valuable review clearly outlines the unmet needs in paediatric psychopharmacology. The most critical unmet needs today in paediatric psychopharmacology include but are not limited to the off-label use of medication and the need of preclinical data to increase the chance for the successful development of targeted and innovative therapeutics (for a complete overview, please see Persico et al., 2015).

Pharmacological treatment for child and adolescent mental disorders is limited, and many medications prescribed to paediatric patients are unlicensed and thereby represents off-label use. A large proportion of pharmacological treatment used in youth has indeed solely been studied in adults and often in the context of a different indication (Conroy et al., 2000). Approval in the paediatric indication represents a greater challenge compared with adults due to ethical barriers for performing trials in youth and requiring suitable formulations and extensive long-term data. These challenges with the approval of paediatric pharmacological treatments lead to delays in making a novel treatment option available for youth, and thus often off-label use is initiated in daily clinical practice. Across the globe, differences in psychotropic medication prescriptions in children and adolescents (often off label) have been documented among prescribers. In Canada, general practitioners are more likely to prescribe antipsychotic medication compared with psychiatrists (Murphy et al., 2013), while in Germany, hospital-based specialists prescribe a higher number of off-label antidepressant medication compared with general practitioners (Dörks et al., 2013). Importantly, while children and adolescents are in need of novel and innovative treatment options to improve their lives, there is a need for substantiating the use of the pharmacological treatment with regulatory approval and long-term efficacy and safety data.

A further primary unmet focus point identified in child and adolescent psychopharmacology is the need for improved preclinical data to increase the chance for the successful development of targeted and innovative therapeutics. Vital preclinical approaches providing potential new avenues include genetics, animal models, stem cells, and RNA-based therapeutics. In the last decades, research has seen a surge in progress towards understanding the genetic underpinning of child and adolescent psychopathology. A multitude of genes has today been identified exerting disease risk in various psychiatric disorders (Vorstman and Ophoff, 2013; Jeste and Geschwind, 2014; Topper et al., 2011). Importantly the large number of identified risk genes in psychiatric disorders converge on a handful of biological pathways (Persico and Napolioni, 2013; De Rubeis et al., 2014; Pinto et al., 2014), thus providing not only insight into the neurobiology of disease but opening new avenues for treatment options. Bioinformatics aimed at defining functional gene networks underlying diseases in addition to novel experimental approaches based on pluripotent stem cells (Kitchener and Wu, 2015; Yamanaka, 2008), and RNA-based approaches (van deVondervoort et al., 2013; Meng et al., 2015) offer great potential for innovation in psychiatry. Lastly, advances in genetic and experimental approaches are complemented with evaluation in animal models. Animal models have played a crucial role in the advancement of the field of psychopharmacology and have throughout the years generated a wealth of knowledge pertaining to neuroanatomy, neurochemistry, and behaviour. However, animal models indeed do not reproduce human conditions. Assuming the latter and projecting human traits onto animals has also hindered preclinical assessment due to the lack of translatability and thereby leading to failures (Kas et al., 2014). Instead, animal models in conjunction with assays offer great value for tapping into specific symptoms present in human conditions based on the cross-species translational knowledge at both the behavioural and neurobiological levels.

5.6 Translational disease platform

Translational clinical-preclinical disease platform establishment is vital for the purpose of innovative pharmacological treatment development based on the unmet needs of a patient population. A disease platform represents a foundation which links the knowledge from the clinic to the neurobiological underpinning of a disease. To improve the quality of life of patients living with mental disorders, we need not only to improve the overall symptomatology but also to uncover remaining unmet needs interlinked with functioning. For example, in ADHD, pharmacological agents have been demonstrated to improve symptomatology as measured with the accepted clinical rating scales. That said, digging deeper into the symptomatology, we uncover that it is made up of triage of symptoms with each differentially affected by the varied pharmacological options available to ADHD patients. In ADHD the core domains which are afflicted are (a) cognition, (b) impulsivity, and (c) hyperactivity. ADHD patients will exhibit various levels of deficits in any of the three domains, which also will likely change throughout the lifespan. The typical picture of an ADHD child is that of the boy who is excessively hyperactive and unable to sit still 'climbing' up the walls. Today, however, the increased knowledge has culminated in the understanding that ADHD can manifest in many different ways including a child who is inattentive and impulsive without signs of hyperactivity, who will early on show signs of academic challenges, low self-esteem, and difficulties with social interactions. Furthermore a hyperactive child can in adulthood manifest deficits primarily in the context of executive function deficits and impulse control, which then are interlinked with occupational challenges and low self-esteem, family disturbances, accidents, and substance abuse. These examples depict the complexity of managing ADHD patients who are clearly a heterogeneous population. ADHD does not stand alone in this – all child and adolescent mental disorders represent a complex and heterogeneous population.

To support patients based on their individual needs, we propose to start with an in-depth understanding of the core domains and with the establishment of the treatment effects within each as well as the unmet needs within each. Sikirica and colleagues described remaining needs in ADHD patients following pharmacological treatment per core domain based on insights from both adolescent patients and caregivers (Sikirica et al., 2015). The data clearly highlight that while pharmacological treatment is beneficial, many challenges remain in inattention, hyperactivity, and impulsivity.

The translational platform establishment is initiated by the clinical evaluation per core domain. Imaging studies during the performance of attentional and impulsivity tasks have demonstrated the engagement of the frontostriatal networks with hypoactivation of the network in ADHD patients compared with controls (Hart et al., 2013; Rubia et al., 2014). Thus imaging data have depicted the connection between the behaviours of attention and impulsivity in the clinic with the underlying biological circuitry. Importantly to develop novel therapeutic options, it is vital to create the understanding of the behaviour and biological underpinning in the preclinical setting. Translation at the biological level is more direct compared with translation at the behavioural level between humans and mice/rats as long as the target and underlying mechanism are conserved between the species. Indeed, Robbins and colleagues have conducted a series of elegant lesion studies, which have culminated in a map of behavioural aspects of attention and impulsivity and the underlying regions/networks involved in addition to the role of the neurotransmitter systems (Bari and Robbins, 2011). The lesion studies in the preclinical setting depict evidence of frontostriatal network engagement in attention and impulsivity in alignment with the clinical imaging data. Thus, in conclusion, attention and impulsivity behaviours are present both in the clinic and in the preclinical setting with the underlying frontostriatal involvement being documented in both humans and animals.

To increase the chance of successfully developing a novel, innovative agent improving aspects of inattention and impulsivity, it is vital to identify assays which are comparable clinically and preclinically regarding not only the behaviours but also the underlying biology. The continuous performance tasks (CPT) is a sensitive detection of deficits in ADHD (Riccio and Reynolds, 2001; Teicher et al., 2004). In the clinic, various versions such as the RVIP, TOVA, and Conners measure attention and inhibitory control (e.g. action impulsivity) objectively. In the computer-based tasks, the patient scans sequences and is required to (a) detect low probability targets and (b) inhibit the response to nontargets. Preclinically, the operant five-choice serial-reaction time task (5CSRT, Carli et al., 1983) is used to measure attention and inhibitory control (e.g. action impulsivity). The test requires that rats/mice (a) detect a target stimulus in a five-hole aperture and (b) inhibit responding prior to target presentation. Both the clinical CPT and the preclinical 5CSRT assays measure aspects of attention and impulsivity, but indeed the clinical and preclinical assessments are not behaviourally equal with primary differences manifested in task performance and motivation effects. Moreover, thus clinical and preclinical evaluation for aspects of attention and impulsivity have demonstrated that the CPT and 5CSRT tasks do indeed measure aspects of the core deficits in ADHD, and importantly imaging and lesion studies have confirmed that in the clinic and the preclinical setting, attentional and impulsivity deficits are linked to the frontostriatal circuitry.

A final key component in the translational platform establishment is the assessment of how currently available and efficacious therapeutics perform in the clinical and preclinical assays for attention and impulsivity. Stimulants are the most frequent treatment option in ADHD with amphetamine and methylphenidate preferentially increasing norepinephrine and dopamine within the prefrontal cortex relative to other cortical and subcortical regions in addition to increasing striatal dopamine levels (Berridge and Devilbiss, 2011). Atomoxetine is the alternative treatment option in ADHD elevating norepinephrine and dopamine levels in the prefrontal cortex (Bymaster et al., 2002; Yamamoto and Novotney, 1998) with minimal effects on striatal dopamine levels (Bymaster et al., 2002). In human subjects, methylphenidate has been shown to improve sustained attention in both ADHD patients and healthy controls with a low level of baseline performance (Turner et al., 2005; del Campo et al., 2013), while atomoxetine improves response inhibition (Gau and Shang, 2010; Chamberlain et al., 2007). Preclinically, data in the 5CSRT task have demonstrated that stimulant improvements in choice accuracy are difficult to consistently demonstrate (Navarra et al., 2008), which could however be improved by optimising the paradigm to focus on 'poor performing' rats (Puumala et al., 1996) since the attentional improvements in humans are noted in both ADHD and control subjects with low baseline level of performance. In the clinic, atomoxetine is shown to improve response inhibition which is also demonstrated preclinically via dose-dependent decreases in premature responses in the 5CSRT (Navarra et al., 2008; Baarendse and Vanderschuren, 2012). Just as noted on the value of evaluating 'poor performing' rats in terms of attentional tasks, studying pharmacological effects in impulsive rats can be of great value. Impulsive rats represent 10% of the naturally occurring phenotype with stable and persistent expression throughout adulthood (Robinson et al., 2009). These impulsive rats exhibit a selective deficit in premature response in the 5CSRT task while showing no difference in further behavioural readouts (Dalley et al., 2008; Blondeau and Dellu-Hagedorn, 2007; Puumala et al., 1996). Atomoxetine has been demonstrated to attenuate the impulsive phenotype (Blondeau and Dellu-Hagedorn, 2007) in line with the clinical findings on action impulsivity.

Impulsivity in ADHD is marked by either action impulsivity (measured in CPT and 5CSRT tasks) or choice impulsivity (measured with the delayed discounting task (DDT) clinically and preclinically). DDT deficits have been observed in ADHD patients (Sonuga-Barke et al., 1992). Additionally, teachers' rating of impulsivity and hyperactivity predicts delay aversion (Solanto et al., 2001). The clinical version of the DDT is either hypothetical (Green and Myerson, 2004) or real time (Reynolds and Schiffbauer, 2004) measuring delayed discounting. Preclinically the DDT is either a T maze task in juvenile rats or an operant task testing low and high impulsive rats. Again similar to the CPT/5CSRT, the clinical and preclinical DDT tasks while measuring aspects of choice impulsivity are not behaviourally equal with differences in task performance and motivation effects. Imaging studies have revealed that delay discounting involves the brain reward circuits linking the ventral striatum to frontal regions (McClure et al., 2004; Sonuga-Barke et al., 2008). Lesion studies in rats have allowed for a detailed map out of the brain regions underlying choice impulsivity (Winstanley et al., 2006; Cardinal et al., 2001) pointing to the frontostriatal involvement in line with the clinical findings. The pharmacological effect of methylphenidate has been tested in the human DDT model and is shown to demonstrate improvements in choice impulsivity (Shiels et al., 2009). ADHD therapeutics in the rodent T maze version of the task is shown to improve choice impulsivity albeit in a narrow dose range (Bizot et al., 2011), and in the operant version, stimulants are shown to improve choice impulsivity. In conclusion, while ADHD therapeutics improves impulsivity, a dissection of impulsivity points towards stimulant improvement in choice versus atomoxetine improvement in action impulsivity based on the preclinical evaluations.

The granular evaluation of pharmacological agents in the clinical and preclinical settings may not only uncover differential effects of current medication but open avenues for next-generation precision-based treatment options.

5.7 Conclusion

Psychopharmacological management of children and adolescents is critical for the improvements in functioning and the support of optimal life quality. Treatment options available today ameliorate patients' lives but do not fully extinguish the challenges faced by each individual patient.

In all child and adolescent mental disorders, it is vital to move the frontiers of science and technology for the development of innovative precision-based pharmacological treatment and their combination with novel approaches to child and adolescent management. Advances in 'digital therapies' offer new avenues where technological advances pose options not available to us in the past. An example of digital technology is neurofeedback via feedback slowly altering the brain by modulating electrical signals which then results in behavioural changes. The latest systematic review of neurofeedback based on metaanalysis in children concluded that neurofeedback had a more durable treatment effect lasting at least 6 months in comparison with nonactive control (Van Doren et al., 2019). In conclusion, novel nonpharmacological treatment options may offer potential additional benefits for youth and thereby add to the management of psychiatric diseases.

Importantly the achievement of optimal quality of life requires that innovative scientific and technological advances be blended into a multidimensional treatment paradigm involving healthcare professionals, family members, teachers, and psychosocial workers to create a holistic solution based on the unique needs of the individual patient.

References

Adesman, A.R., 2001. The diagnosis and management of attention-deficit/hyperactivity disorder in pediatric patients. Prim. Care Companion J. Clin. Psychiatry. 3 (2), 66–77.
Arango, C., 2015. Present and future of developmental neuropsy-chopharmacology. Eur. Neuropsychopharmacol. 25 (5), 703–712.
Baarendse, P.J., Vanderschuren, L.J., 2012. Dissociable effects of monoamine reuptake inhibitors on distinct forms of impulsive behavior in rats. Psychopharmacology 219 (2), 313–326.
Bari, A., Robbins, T.W., 2011. Animal models of ADHD. Curr. Top. Behav. Neurosci. 7, 149–185.
Barkley, R.A., Fischer, M., Smallish, L., Fletcher, K., 2004. Young adult follow-up of hyperactive children: antisocial activities and drug use. J. Child Psychol. Psychiatry 45 (2), 195–211.
Berridge, C.W., Devilbiss, D.M., 2011. Psychostimulants as cognitive enhancers: the prefrontal cortex, catecholamines, and attention-deficit/hyperactivity disorder. Biol. Psychiatry 69 (12), e101–e111.
Biederman, J., Monuteaux, M.C., Spencer, T., 2008. Stimulant therapy and risk for subsequent substance use disorders in male adults with ADHD: a naturalistic controlled 10-year follow-up study. Am. J. Psychiatr. 165, 597–603.
Bizot, J.C., David, S., Trovero, F., 2011. Effects of atomoxetine, desipramine, d-amphetamine and methylphenidate on impulsivity in juvenile rats, measured in a T-maze procedure. Neurosci. Lett. 489 (1), 20–24.
Blondeau, C., Dellu-Hagedorn, F., 2007. Dimensional analysis of ADHD subtypes in rats. Biol. Psychiatry 61 (12), 1340–1350.
Bradley, C., 1937. The Behaviour of Children Receiving Benzedrine. Amercian Psychiatric Association, pp. 577–585.

Bymaster, F.P., Katner, J.S., Nelson, D.L., Hemrick-Luecke, S.K., Threlkeld, P.G., Heiligenstein, J.H., Morin, S.M., Gehlert, D.R., Perry, K.W., 2002. Atomoxetine increases extracellular levels of norepinephrine and dopamine in prefrontal cortex of rat: a potential mechanism for efficacy in attention deficit/hyperactivity disorder. Neuropsychopharmacology 27 (5), 699–711.

Cardinal, R.N., Pennicott, D.R., Sugathapala, C.L., Robbins, T.W., Everitt, B.J., 2001. Impulsive choice induced in rats by lesions of the nucleus accumbens core. Science 292 (5526), 2499–2501.

Carli, M., Robbins, T.W., Evenden, J.L., Everitt, B.J., 1983. Effects of lesions to ascending noradrenergic neurones on performance of a 5-choice serial reaction task in rats; implications for theories of dorsal noradrenergic bundle function based on selective attention and arousal. Behav. Brain Res. 9 (3), 361–380.

Chamberlain, S.R., Del Campo, N., Dowson, J., Müller, U., Clark, L., Robbins, T.W., Sahakian, B.J., 2007. Atomoxetine improved response inhibition in adults with attention deficit/hyperactivity disorder. Biol. Psychiatry 62 (9), 977–984.

Conroy, S., Choonara, I., Impicciatore, P., Mohn, A., Arnell, H., Rane, A., Knoeppel, C., Seyberth, H., Pandolfini, C., Raffaelli, M.P., Rocchi, F., Bonati, M., Jong, G., de Hoog, M., van den Anker, J., 2000. Survey of unlicensed and off label drug use in paediatric wards in European countries. European Network for Drug Investigation in Children. BMJ 320 (7227), 79–82.

Costello, E.J., Copeland, W., Angold, A., 2011. Trends in psychopathology across the adolescent years: what changes when children become adolescents, and when adolescents become adults? J. Child Psychol. Psychiatry 52, 1015–1025.

Dalley, J.W., Mar, A.C., Economidou, D., Robbins, T.W., 2008. Neurobehavioral mechanisms of impulsivity: fronto-striatal systems and functional neurochemistry. Pharmacol. Biochem. Behav. 90 (2), 250–260.

De Rubeis, S., He, X., Goldberg, A.P., Poultney, C.S., Samocha, K., Cicek, A.E., Kou, Y., Liu, L., Fromer, M., Walker, S., Singh, T., Klei, L., Kosmicki, J., Shih-Chen, F., Aleksic, B., Biscaldi, M., Bolton, P.F., Brownfeld, J.M., Cai, J., Campbell, N.G., Carracedo, A., Chahrour, M.H., Chiocchetti, A.G., Coon, H., Crawford, E.L., Curran, S.R., Dawson, G., Duketis, E., Fernandez, B.A., Gallagher, L., Geller, E., Guter, S.J., Hill, R.S., Ionita-Laza, J., Jimenz Gonzalez, P., Kilpinen, H., Klauck, S.M., Kolevzon, A., Lee, I., Lei, I., Lei, J., Lehtimäki, T., Lin, C.F., Ma'ayan, A., Marshall, C.R., McInnes, A.L., Neale, B., Owen, M.J., Ozaki, N., Parellada, M., Parr, J.R., Purcell, S., Puura, K., Rajagopalan, D., Rehnström, K., Reichenberg, A., Sabo, A., Sachse, M., Sanders, S.J., Schafer, C., Schulte-Rüther, M., Skuse, D., Stevens, C., Szatmari, P., Tammimies, K., Valladares, O., Voran, A., Li-San, W., Weiss, L.A., Willsey, A.J., Yu, T.W., Yuen, R.K.DDD StudyHomozygosity Mapping Collaborative for AutismUK 10K ConsortiumCook, E.H., Freitag, C.M., Gill, M., Hultman, C.M., Lehner, T., Palotie, A., Schellenberg, G.D., Sklar, P., State, M.W., Sutcliffe, J.S., Walsh, C.A., Scherer, S.W., Zwick, M.E., Barett, J.C., Cutler, D.J., Roeder, K., Devlin, B., Daly, M.J., Buxbaum, J.D., 2014. Synaptic, transcriptional and chromatin genes disrupted in autism. Nature 515 (7526), 209–215.

del Campo, N., Fryer, T.D., Hong, Y.T., Smith, R., Brichard, L., Acosta-Cabronero, J., Chamberlain, S.R., Tait, R., Izquierdo, D., Regenthal, R., Dowson, J., Suckling, J., Baron, J.C., Aigbirhio, F.I., Robbins, T.W., Sahakian, B.J., Müller, U., 2013. A positron emission tomography study of nigro-striatal dopaminergic mechanisms underlying attention: implications for ADHD and its treatment. Brain 136 (Pt 11), 3252–3270.

Dörks, M., Langner, I., Dittmann, U., Timmer, A., Garbe, E., 2013. Antidepressant drug use and off-label prescribing in children and adolescents in Germany: results from a large population-based cohort study. Eur. Child Adolesc. Psychiatry 22 (8), 511–518.

Ekman, J.T., Gustafsson, P.A., 2000. Stimulants in AD/HD, a controversial treatment only in Sweden? Eur. Child Adolesc. Psychiatry 9 (4), 312–313.

Faraone, S.V., Glatt, S.J., 2010. A comparison of the efficacy of medications for adult attention-deficit/hyperactivity disorder using meta-analysis of effect sizes. J. Clin. Psychiatry 71 (6).

Fegert, J.M., Kolch, M., Zito, J.M., 2006. Antidepressant use in children and adolescents in Germany. J. Child Adolesc. Psychopharmacol. 16, 197–206.

Gau, S.S., Shang, C.Y., 2010. Improvement of executive functions in boys with attention deficit hyperactivity disorder: an open-label follow-up study with once-daily atomoxetine. Int. J. Neuropsychopharmacol. 13 (2), 243–256.

Gjervan, B., Torgersen, T., Nordahl, H.M., Rasmussen, K., 2012. Functional impairment and occupational outcome in adults with ADHD. J. Atten. Disord. 16 (7), 544–552.

Goldman, L.S., Genel, M., Bezman, R.J., Slanetz, P.J., 1998. Diagnosis and treatment of attention-deficit/hyperactivity disorder in children and adolescents. Council on Scientific Affairs, American Medical Association. JAMA 279 (14), 1100–1107.

Green, L., Myerson, J., 2004. A discounting framework for choice with delayed and probabilistic rewards. Psychol. Bull. 130 (5), 769–792. Review.

Greenhill, L.L., Abikoff, H., Chuang, S., 2006. Efficacy and safety of immediate-release methylphenidate treatment for preschoolers with ADHD. J. Am. Acad. Child Adolesc. Psychiatry 45, 1284–1293.

Hart, H., Radua, J., Nakao, T., Mataix-Cols, D., Rubia, K., 2013. Meta-analysis of functional magnetic resonance imaging studies of inhibition and attention in attention-deficit/hyperactivity disorder: exploring task-specific, stimulant medication, and age effects. JAMA Psychiatry 70 (2), 185–198.

Jensen, P.S., Kettle, L., Roper, M.T., Sloan, M.T., Dulcan, M.K., Hoven, C., Bird, H.R., Bauermeister, J.J., Payne, J.D., 1999. Are stimulants overprescribed? Treatment of ADHD in four US communities. J. Am. Acad. Child Adolesc. Psychiatry 38 (7), 797–804.

Jensen, P.S., Goldman, E., Offord, D., Costello, E.J., Friedman, R., Huff, B., Crowe, M., Amsel, L., Bennett, K., Bird, H., Conger, R., Fisher, P., Hoagwood, K., Kessler, R.C., Roberts, R., 2011. Overlooked and underserved: "action signs" for identifying children with unmet mental health needs. Pediatrics 128, 970–979.

Jeste, S.S., Geschwind, D.H., 2014. Disentangling the heterogeneity of autism spectrum disorder through genetic findings. Nat. Rev. Neurol. 10 (2), 74–81.

Kas, M.J., Glennon, J.C., Buitelaar, J., Ey, E., Biemans, B., Crawley, J., Ring, R.H., Lajonchere, C., Esclassan, F., Talpos, J., Noldus, L.P., Burbach, J.P., Steckler, T., 2014. Assessing behavioural and cognitive domains of autism spectrum disorders in rodents: current status and future perspectives. Psychopharmacology 231 (6), 1125–1146.

Kennard, B.D., Silva, S., Vitiello, B., 2006. Remission and residual symptoms after acute treatment of adolescents with major depressive disorder. J. Am. Acad. Child Adolesc. Psychiatry 45, 1404–1411.

Kieling, C., Baker-Henningham, H., Belfer, M., Conti, G., Ertem, I., Omigbodun, O., Rohde, L.A., Srinath, S., Ulkuer, N., Rahman, A., 2011. Child and adolescent mental health worldwide: evidence for action. Lancet 378, 1515–1525.

Kitchener, D.W., Wu, J.C., 2015. Induced pluripotent stem cells. JAMA 313 (16), 1613–1614.

Kociancic, T., Reed, M.D., Findling, R.L., 2004. Evaluation of risks associated with short- and long-term psychostimulant therapy for treatment of ADHD in children. Expert Opin. Drug Saf. 3 (2), 93–100.

Lichtenstein, P., Halldner, L., Zetterqvist, J., Sjölander, A., Serlachius, E., Fazel, S., Långström, N., Larsson, H., 2012. Medication for attention deficit-hyperactivity disorder and criminality. N. Engl J. Med. 367 (21), 2006–2014.

Llana, M.E., Crismon, M.L., 1999. Methylphenidate: increased abuse or appropriate use? J. Am. Pharm. Assoc. (Wash.) 39 (4), 526–530.

McClure, S.M., Laibson, D.I., Loewenstein, G., Cohen, J.D., 2004. Separate neural systems value immediate and delayed monetary rewards. Science 306 (5695), 503–507.

Meng, L., Ward, A.J., Chun, S., Bennett, C.F., Beaudet, A.L., Rigo, F., 2015. Towards a therapy for Angelman syndrome by targeting a long non-coding RNA. Nature 518 (7539), 409–412.

Murphy, A.L., Gardner, D.M., Cooke, C., Kisely, S., Hughes, J., Kutcher, S.P., 2013. Prescribing trends of antipsychotics in youth receiving income assistance: results from a retrospective population database study. BMC Psychiatry 13, 198.

Navarra, R., Graf, R., Huang, Y., Logue, S., Comery, T., Hughes, Z., Day, M., 2008. Effects of atomoxetine and methylphenidate on attention and impulsivity in the 5-choice serial reaction time test. Prog. Neuro-Psychopharmacol. Biol. Psychiatry 32 (1), 34–41.

Naveed, S., Waqas, A., Majeed, S., Zeshan, M., Jahan, N., Sheikh, M.H., 2017. Child psychiatry: a scientometric analysis 1980-2016. F1000Res. 6, 1293.

Olfson, M., Blanco, C., Wang, S., Laje, G., Correll, C.U., 2014. National trends in the mental healthcare of children, adolescents, and adults by office-based physicians. JAMA Psychiatry 71, 81–90.

Persico, A.M., Napolioni, V., 2013. Autism genetics. Behav. Brain Res. 251, 95–112.

Persico, A.M., Arango, C., Buitelaar, J.K., Correll, C.U., Glennon, J.C., Hoekstra, P.J., Moreno, C., Vitiello, B., Vorstman, J., Zuddas, A., European Child and Adolescent Clinical Psychopharmacology Network, 2015. Unmet needs in paediatric psychopharmacology: present scenario and future perspectives. Eur. Neuropsychopharmacol. 25 (10), 1513–1531.

Pinto, D., Delaby, E., Merico, D., Barbosa, M., Merikangas, A., Klei, L., Thiruvahindrapuram, B., Xu, X., Ziman, R., Wang, Z., Vorstman, J.A., Thompson, A., Regan, R., Pilorge, M., Pellecchia, G., Pagnamenta, A.T., Oliveira, B., Marshall, C.R., Magalhaes, T.R., Lowe, J.K., Howe, J.L., Griswold, A.J., Gilbert, J., Duketis, E., Dombroski, B.A., DeJonge, M.V., Cuccaro, M., Crawford, E.L., Correia, C.T., Conroy, J., Conceição, I.C., Chiocchetti, A.G., Casey, J.P., Cai, G., Cabrol, C., Bolshakova, N., Bacchelli, E., Anney, R., Gallinger, S., Cotterchio, M., Casey, G., Zwaigenbaum, L., Wittemeyer, K., Wing, K., Wallace, S., van Engeland, H., Tryfon, A., Thomson, S., Soorya, L., Rogé, B., Roberts, W., Poustka, F., Mouga, S., Minshew, N., McInnes, L.A., McGrew, S.G., Lord, C., Leboyer, M., LeCouteur, A.S., Kolevzon, A., Jiménez González, P., Jacob, S., Holt, R., Guter, S., Green, J., Green, A., Gillberg, C., Fernandez, B.A., Duque, F., Delorme, R., Dawson, G., Chaste, P., Café, C., Brennan, S., Bourgeron, T., Bolton, P.F., Bölte, S., Bernier, R., Baird, G., Bailey, A.J., Anagnostou, E., Almeida, J., Wijsman, E.M., Vieland, V.J., Vicente, A.M., Schellenberg, G.D., Pericak-Vance, M., Paterson, A.D., Parr, J.R., Oliveira, G., Nurnberger, J.I., Monaco, A.P., Maestrini, E., Klauck, S.M., Hakonarson, H., Haines, J.L., Geschwind, D.H., Freitag, C.M., Folstein, S.E., Ennis, S., Coon, H., Battaglia, A., Szatmari, P., Sutcliffe, J.S., Hallmayer, J., Gill, M., Cook, E.H., Buxbaum, J.D., Devlin, B., Gallagher, L., Betancur, C., Scherer, S.W., 2014. Convergence of genes and cellular pathways dysregulated in autism spectrum disorders. Am. J. Hum. Genet. 94 (5), 677–694.

Puumala, T., Ruotsalainen, S., Jäkälä, P., Koivisto, E., Riekkinen Jr., P., Sirviö, J., 1996. Behavioral and pharmacological studies on the validation of a new animal model for attention deficit hyperactivity disorder. Neurobiol. Learn. Mem. 66 (2), 198–211.

Rani, F., Murray, M.L., Byrne, P.J., Wong, I.C., 2008. Epidemiologic features of antipsychotic prescribing to children and adolescents in primary care in the United Kingdom. Pediatrics 121, 1002–1009.

Rey, J.M., Assumpção Jr., F.B., Bernad, C.A., 2015. History of Child Psychiatry. IACAPAP Textbook of Child and Adolescent Mental Health. 1–72.

Reynolds, B., Schiffbauer, R., 2004. Measuring state changes in human delay discounting: an experiential discounting task. Behav. Processes 67 (3), 343–356.

Rho, J.M., Storey, T.W., 2001. Molecular ontogeny of major neurotransmitter receptor systems in the mammalian central nervous system: norepinephrine, dopamine, serotonin, acetylcholine, and glycine. J. Child Neurol. 16, 271–279.

Riccio, C.A., Reynolds, C.R., 2001. Continuous performance tests are sensitive to ADHD in adults but lack specificity. A review and critique for differential diagnosis. Ann. N. Y. Acad. Sci. 931, 113–139. Review.

Robinson, E.S., Eagle, D.M., Economidou, D., Theobald, D.E., Mar, A.C., Murphy, E.R., Robbins, T.W., Dalley, J.W., 2009. Behavioural characterisation of high impulsivity on the 5-choice serial reaction time task: specific deficits in 'waiting' versus 'stopping'. Behav. Brain Res. 196 (2), 310–316.

Rubia, K., Alegria, A.A., Cubillo, A.I., Smith, A.B., Brammer, M.J., Radua, J., 2014. Effects of stimulants on brain function in attention-deficit/hyperactivity disorder: a systematic review and meta-analysis. Biol. Psychiatry 76 (8), 616–628.

Shiels, K., Hawk, L.W., Reynolds, B., Mazzullo, R.J., Rhodes, J.D., Pelham, W.E., Waxmonsky, J.G., Gangloff, B.P., 2009. Effects of methylphenidate on discounting of delayed rewards in attention deficit/hyperactivity disorder. Exp. Clin. Psychopharmacol. 17 (5), 291–301.

Sikirica, V., Flood, E., Dietrich, C.N., Quintero, J., Harpin, V., Hodgkins, P., Skrodzki, K., Beusterien, K., Erder, M.H., 2015. Unmet needs associated with attention-deficit/hyperactivity disorder in eight European countries as reported by caregivers and adolescents: results from qualitative research. Patient 8 (3), 269–281.

Solanto, M.V., Abikoff, H., Sonuga-Barke, E., Schachar, R., Logan, G.D., Wigal, T., Hechtman, L., Hinshaw, S., Turkel, E., 2001. The ecological validity of delay aversion and response inhibition as measures of impulsivity in AD/HD: a supplement to the NIMH multimodal treatment study of AD/HD. J. Abnorm. Child Psychol. 29 (3), 215–228.

Sonuga-Barke, E.J., Taylor, E., Heptinstall, E., 1992. Hyperactivity and delay aversion—II. The effect of self versus externally imposed stimulus presentation periods on memory. J. Child Psychol. Psychiatry 33 (2), 399–409.

Sonuga-Barke, E.J., Sergeant, J.A., Nigg, J., Willcutt, E., 2008. Executive dysfunction and delay aversion in attention deficit hyperactivity disorder: nosologic and diagnostic implications. Child Adolesc. Psychiatr. Clin. N. Am. 17 (2), 367–384. ix.

Swanson, J.M., Kraemer, H.C., Hinshaw, S.P., 2001. Clinical relevance of the primary findings of the MTA: success rate based on severity of ADHD and ODD symptoms at the end of treatment. J. Am. Acad. Child Adolesc. Psychiatry 40, 168–179.

Teicher, M.H., Lowen, S.B., Polcari, A., Foley, M., McGreenery, C.E., 2004. Novel strategy for the analysis of CPT data provides new insight into the effects of methylphenidate on attentional states in children with ADHD. J. Child Adolesc. Psychopharmacol. 14 (2), 219–232.

Topper, S., Ober, C., Das, S., 2011. Exome sequencing and the genetics of intellectual disability. Clin. Genet. 80 (2), 117–126.

Turner, D.C., Blackwell, A.D., Dowson, J.H., McLean, A., Sahakian, B.J., 2005. Neurocognitive effects of methylphenidate in adult attention-deficit/hyperactivity disorder. Psychopharmacology 178 (2-3), 286–295.

van deVondervoort, I.I., Gordebeke, P.M., Khoshab, N., Tiesinga, P.H., Buitelaar, J.K., Kozicz, T., Aschrafi, A., Glennon, J.C., 2013. Long non-coding RNAs in neurodevelopmental disorders. Front. Mol. Neurosci. 6, 53.

Van Doren, J., Arns, M., Heinrich, H., Vollebregt, M.A., Strehl, U., K Loo, S., 2019. Sustained effects of neurofeedback in ADHD: a systematic review and meta-analysis. Eur. Child Adolesc. Psychiatry 28 (3), 293–305. https://doi.org/10.1007/s00787-018-1121-4.

Vitiello, B., 2008. An international perspective on pediatric psychopharmacology. Int. Rev. Psychiatry 20, 121–126.

Vitiello, B., Rohde, P., Silva, S.G., 2006. Effects of treatment on level of functioning, global health, and quality of life in depressed adolescents. J. Am. Acad. Child Adolesc. Psychiatry 45, 1419–1426.

Vorstman, J.A., Ophoff, R.A., 2013. Genetic causes of developmental disorders. Curr. Opin. Neurol. 26 (2), 128–136.

WHO, 1975. World Health Organization: Technical Report Series. WHO, Geneva.

WHO, 2016. World Health Organization: Technical Report Series. WHO, Geneva.

Wilens, T.E., Adamson, J., Monuteaux, M.C., 2008. Effect of prior stimulant treatment for attention-deficit/hyperactivity disorder on subsequent risk for cigarette smoking and alcohol and drug use disorders in adolescents. Arch. Pediatr. Adolesc. Med. 162, 916–921.

Winstanley, C.A., Eagle, D.M., Robbins, T.W., 2006. Behavioral models of impulsivity in relation to ADHD: translation between clinical and preclinical studies. Clin. Psychol. Rev. 26 (4), 379–395.

Yamamoto, B.K., Novotney, S., 1998. Regulation of extracellular dopamine by the norepinephrine transporter. J. Neurochem. 71 (1), 274–280.

Yamanaka, S., 2008. Induction of pluripotent stem cells from mouse fibroblasts by four transcriptionfactors. Cell Prolif. 41 (Suppl.1), 51–56.

Ethical aspects of research in paediatric psychopharmacology

Philippe Auby[a], Jelena Ivkovic[b]
[a]Otsuka Pharmaceutical Development & Commercialisation Europe, Frankfurt am Main, Germany, [b]Senior Medical Specialist, Early Psychiatry Projects, H. Lundbeck A/S, Copenhagen, Denmark

> *The pediatric population represents a vulnerable subgroup. Therefore, special measures are needed to protect the rights of pediatric study participants and to shield them from undue risk.*
>
> **ICH E11**

6.1 Introduction

Despite worldwide societal increase pressure to get children behaving like adults, with the debates around the complicated topic of whether juveniles should be charged as adults in the criminal justice system, paediatric patients do represent a vulnerable population. Triggered by US and EU paediatric regulations, more studies in paediatric patients are anticipated to be conducted. Such increase emphasises the necessity to avoid children facing undue risks of pain and harm. In this chapter, we will discuss common paediatric considerations and specific aspects of child and adolescent psychopharmacology research 'because of the ethical issues surrounding research in what is in effect a doubly vulnerable group of individuals' (Tan and Koelch, 2008). Medical research has a horrible dark history, and physicians and researchers have repetitively violated the rights of human beings. Per nature, ethics is an evolving field. With the worldwide paediatric regulations evidencing a current societal shift from protecting children against clinical research to a new emerging paradigm of protecting children through clinical research, more research is anticipated. Therefore taking into account that each paediatric research is different and unique, our objective is to bring a conceptual perspective rather than provide an ethical checklist. Specific considerations on paediatric psychopharmacology will also be discussed.

6.2 Historical perspective on ethics

Primum non nocere

It is crucial to emphasise this fundamental ethical principle, 'First do no harm'. Often wrongly attributed to the Hippocratic Oath, however, in line with the major ethical principles of the Oath, these simple words remind us that medical research has a horrible dark history and that the rights of human beings have been repetitively violated by physicians regardless of the Hippocratic Oath or ethical standards. 'Primum non nocere' is all but a literal statement. It is a quite subtle way to remind all health care professionals that they always must balance the risks versus the benefits for any research, diagnostic, or therapeutic procedures. In line with such interpretation of 'primum non nocere', ICH-E11 (R1) states: 'Without a prospect of direct clinical benefit from an experimental intervention or procedure, the foreseeable risks and burdens to which pediatric participants would be exposed must be low, i.e., comparable to those risks and burdens encountered in their routine clinical care'.

We also strongly advocate that patients or research subjects should systematically be associated with such a decision-making process. Ultimately, 'primum non nocere' is also a reminder that physicians should neither overestimate their capacity to heal nor underestimate their capacity to cause harm.

Medical research has a horrible dark history. 'Dark Medicine: Rationalizing Unethical Medical Research' published in 2007 reported the outcome of a 2004 interdisciplinary conference at the University of Pennsylvania, presenting, in particular, some cases of unethical research in Japan, the United States, and Germany. Sixteen texts are examining World War II crimes, postwar issues, and present-day challenges (LaFleur et al., 2007). LaFleur emphasises the need to learn from the past: 'The focus of this volume is not so much on the history of the episodes of dark medical research... as it is on how much research was rationalized – precisely because the patterns of rationalization are more likely to show up again in our own time than are the specifics of past actions'.

The case of Unit 731, a covert biological and chemical warfare research and development unit of the Imperial Japanese Army that undertook lethal human experimentation during the Second Sino-Japanese War (1937–45) of World War II, is detailed. Unit 731 is responsible for some of the worst war crimes ever committed in the name of science. The researchers involved in these crimes have never been tried. In 2018 the names of thousands of members of Unit 731 were disclosed by the Japanese authorities, in response to a request by Katsuo Nishiyama, a professor at Shiga University of Medical Science, potentially paving the path for new historical researches.

The Nuremberg Code, which is considered as an essential step in the development of contemporary ethics of medical research, was written in response to the unthinkable atrocities performed by the Nazis in the name of medical science, in direct link with the subsequent Nuremberg trials at the end of World War II in 1947. This 10-point document calls for principles for human experimentation such as informed consent and absence of coercion, properly formulated scientific experimentations, and permanent need to balance risks/benefits to the subjects (Table 6.1 – https://history.nih.gov/research/downloads/nuremberg.pdf).

The Nuremberg Code, Declaration of Helsinki, and Declaration of Geneva provide a set of ethical principles regarding human experimentation and clinical care (https://sites.jamanetwork.com/research-ethics/index.html).

The Nuremberg Code, which never passed as a law in any country, still significantly influenced future codes. Interestingly, some criticisms have been made because

Table 6.1 Nuremberg Code

1. The voluntary consent of the human subject is absolutely essential.
   This means that the person involved should have legal capacity to give consent; should be so situated as to be able to exercise free power of choice, without the intervention of any element of force, fraud, deceit, duress, over-reaching, or other ulterior form of constraint or coercion; and should have sufficient knowledge and comprehension of the elements of the subject matter involved, as to enable him to make an understanding and enlightened decision. This latter element requires that, before the acceptance of an affirmative decision by the experimental subject, there should be made known to him the nature, duration, and purpose of the experiment; the method and means by which it is to be conducted; all inconveniences and hazards reasonably to be expected; and the effects upon his health or person, which may possibly come from his participation in the experiment.
   The duty and responsibility for ascertaining the quality of the consent rests upon each individual who initiates, directs or engages in the experiment. It is a personal duty and responsibility which may not be delegated to another with impunity.
2. The experiment should be such as to yield fruitful results for the good of society, unprocurable by other methods or means of study, and not random and unnecessary in nature.
3. The experiment should be so designed and based on the results of animal experimentation and a knowledge of the natural history of the disease or other problem under study, that the anticipated results will justify the performance of the experiment.
4. The experiment should be so conducted as to avoid all unnecessary physical and mental suffering and injury.
5. No experiment should be conducted, where there is an a priori reason to believe that death or disabling injury will occur; except, perhaps, in those experiments where the experimental physicians also serve as subjects.
6. The degree of risk to be taken should never exceed that determined by the humanitarian importance of the problem to be solved by the experiment.
7. Proper preparations should be made and adequate facilities provided to protect the experimental subject against even remote possibilities of injury, disability, or death.
8. The experiment should be conducted only by scientifically qualified persons. The highest degree of skill and care should be required through all stages of the experiment of those who conduct or engage in the experiment.
9. During the course of the experiment, the human subject should be at liberty to bring the experiment to an end, if he has reached the physical or mental state, where continuation of the experiment seemed to him to be impossible.
10. During the course of the experiment, the scientist in charge must be prepared to terminate the experiment at any stage, if he has probable cause to believe, in the exercise of the good faith, superior skill and careful judgement required of him, that a continuation of the experiment is likely to result in injury, disability, or death to the experimental subject.

of its resemblance with the German Guidelines for Human Experimentation of 1931 for 6 of the 10 principles without the authors of the Nuremberg Code making any references to these Guidelines (Ghooi, 2011). Furthermore, these 1931 guidelines, originally published as a Circular of the Reich Minister of the Interior, were not cited during the Nuremberg trial despite the obvious violation of these guidelines by the Nazi physicians. The defendants were charged with war crimes and crimes against humanity as had violated the Hippocratic Oath and behaved in a manner incompatible with their education and profession. The American military tribunal found the tried Nazi doctors guilty of crimes against humanity, and the verdict included a section entitled, 'Permissible Medical Experiments', that is, the Nuremberg Code.

We believe this controversy should not be silenced; however, we tend to disagree with the statement made by Ghooi that the Nuremberg Code 'received far more attention than it ever deserved'. Despite these debates about the code's authorship, scope, and legal standing in both civilian and military science, looking at the evolution of ethics, this 10-point set of rules, developed as an answer to crimes against humanity committed by physicians in concentration camps during World War II, is certainly one of the most influential text in the history of clinical research. The Nuremberg Code has undoubtedly been a milestone in the history of biomedical research ethics (Moreno et al., 2017): 'In a symbolic sense, the Nuremberg Code is part of the infrastructure of the democratic international system that emerged after World War II, with its focus on respect for human rights, individual autonomy, and informed consent. But even that symbolic role is intangible at best. In the field of human research ethics the code was eclipsed by the World Medical Association Declaration of Helsinki in 1964. While the code may have created greater awareness of the importance of human rights in medical science among wide sections of the medical profession, its specific role in international human rights law is modest compared with the 1948 Universal Declaration of Human Rights, created by the United Nations General Assembly in light of 2 world wars'.

The Declaration of Geneva was adopted by the second General Assembly of the World Medical Association (WMA) in Geneva in 1948. It is considered as the contemporary successor to the 2500-year-old Hippocratic Oath, built on its principles. It defines, in a concise way, the professional duties of physicians and affirms the ethical principles of the global medical profession (Parsa-Parsi, 2017). The most notable difference between the Declaration of Geneva and other key ethical documents was determined to be the lack of clear recognition of patient autonomy, despite references to the physician's obligation to exercise respect, beneficence, and medical confidentiality towards his or her patient(s). To address this difference, the following clause was added: 'I WILL RESPECT the autonomy and dignity of my patient'. A few additional changes, including the addition of a subtitle identifying the Declaration as a 'Physician's Pledge', have been performed to enable this critical document to more accurately reflect the challenges and needs of the modern medical profession. 'It is the hope of the World Medical Association that this thorough revision process and follow-up advocacy efforts will lead to more widespread adoption of the Declaration of Geneva on a global scale' (Parsa-Parsi, 2017) (Table 6.2).

Archived previous versions of the Declaration of Geneva can be found on the WMA website.

In 1964 the WMA adopted the Declaration of Helsinki which focuses on the protection of human participants in medical research: 'The "Declaration of Helsinki" by the World Medical Association is a "guide to doctors everywhere" who are

Table 6.2 Declaration of Genova

World Medical Association Declaration of Geneva
The Physician's Pledge
Adopted by the 2nd General Assembly of the World Medical Association, Geneva, Switzerland, September 1948
and amended by the 22nd World Medical Assembly, Sydney, Australia, August 1968
and the 35th World Medical Assembly, Venice, Italy, October 1983
and the 46th WMA General Assembly, Stockholm, Sweden, September 1994
and editorially revised by the 170th WMA Council Session, Divonne-les-Bains, France, May 2005
and the 173rd WMA Council Session, Divonne-les-Bains, France, May 2006
and the WMA General Assembly, Chicago, United States, October 2017
AS A MEMBER OF THE MEDICAL PROFESSION:
I SOLEMNLY PLEDGE to dedicate my life to the service of humanity;
THE HEALTH AND WELL-BEING OF MY PATIENT will be my first consideration;
I WILL RESPECT the autonomy and dignity of my patient;
I WILL MAINTAIN the utmost respect for human life;
I WILL NOT PERMIT considerations of age, disease or disability, creed, ethnic origin, gender, nationality, political affiliation, race, sexual orientation, social standing or any other factor to intervene between my duty and my patient;
I WILL RESPECT the secrets that are confided in me, even after the patient has died;
I WILL PRACTISE my profession with conscience and dignity and in accordance with good medical practice;
I WILL FOSTER the honour and noble traditions of the medical profession;
I WILL GIVE to my teachers, colleagues, and students the respect and gratitude that is their due;
I WILL SHARE my medical knowledge for the benefit of the patient and the advancement of healthcare;
I WILL ATTEND TO my own health, well-being, and abilities in order to provide care of the highest standard;
I WILL NOT USE my medical knowledge to violate human rights and civil liberties, even under threat;
I MAKE THESE PROMISES solemnly, freely, and upon my honour.

---

engaged in clinical research, said Harry S. Gear, MD, WMA secretary-general. Recommendations in the declaration, Gear said, "are offered to all medical men and their colleagues in other disciplines, who undertake scientific and clinical investigations involving human beings. The Declaration of Helsinki is now placed alongside such previous profound documents on professional conduct as the modern form of the Hippocratic Oath, known as the "Declaration of Geneva" and the "International Code of Medical Ethics"'. 'The Declaration of Helsinki was adopted by the 18th World Medical Assembly last June in Helsinki, Finland. Work was started on it following World War II, Gear said' (JAMA, 1964).

The Declaration of Helsinki, despite not being legally binding, is considered as the main pivotal reference about ethics in medical research. It is a true living document that has been revised several times (cf Table 6.3) but has never been exempt from criticism and suggestions for improvement.

Table 6.3 Declaration of Helsinki

Adopted by the 18th WMA General Assembly, Helsinki, Finland, June 1964
Amended by the:
29th WMA General Assembly, Tokyo, Japan, October 1975
35th WMA General Assembly, Venice, Italy, October 1983
41st WMA General Assembly, Hong Kong, September 1989
48th WMA General Assembly, Somerset West, Republic of South Africa, October 1996
52nd WMA General Assembly, Edinburgh, Scotland, October 2000
53rd WMA General Assembly, Washington, DC, USA, October 2002 (Note of Clarification added)
55th WMA General Assembly, Tokyo, Japan, October 2004 (Note of Clarification added)
59th WMA General Assembly, Seoul, Republic of Korea, October 2008
64th WMA General Assembly, Fortaleza, Brazil, October 2013

The influence of the Declaration of Helsinki should not be underestimated. Even if criticised, not used, or even abandoned by some, the Declaration of Helsinki reminds all of us two crucial points:

- First, ethics remains per nature an evolving and complex field.
- Second, declarations, codes, or guidelines will never suffice. Ethics needs active involvement to be continuously enforced and permanently questioned and assessed. 'Science without conscience is but the ruin of the soul', wrote Rabelais, in 1532. The Nazi physicians or the Section 731 members remind us that 'humanity' can be lost.

The 1964 Declaration of Helsinki was a rather short document, focusing on clinical research, interestingly nuancing the first principle of the Nuremberg Code, about voluntary consent. The first revision in 1975 expanded its scope significantly. If the 2000 revision was probably the most controversial, the Declaration of Helsinki was always the subject of important discussions even to long-lasting criticisms.

The last version of 2013 comprises 37 articles.

For more comprehensive information on the Declaration of Helsinki, we recommend the following JAMA webpage: https://sites.jamanetwork.com/research-ethics/index.html.

The American medical community did not fully endorse these three international codes. In a comprehensive article of 2003, called 'Children in Clinical Research: A Conflict of Moral Values', Sharav (2003) explained the origin of the Belmont Report. In 1998, Allen Hornblum observed in his book, Acres of Skin: 'Rather than embracing the Nuremberg Code, the American medical establishment considered it a "good code for barbarians", but an unnecessary code for ordinary physician-scientists'. Then and now, many in the medical research community believed the restrictions imposed by these international codes coupled with the Hippocratic principle were too restrictive for physicians who had not committed medical atrocities… But when revelations surfaced in the press about unethical experiments by American researchers, a national commission was convened, and its 1979 published recommendations, the Belmont Report, laid down three ethical principles to protect human subjects.

The Belmont Report, full title 'The Belmont Report: Ethical Principles and Guidelines for the Protection of Human Subjects of Research, The National Commission for the Protection of Human Subjects of Biomedical and Behavioral

Research', not only is a significant document for research but also is applicable to clinical practice. The primary purpose of the Belmont Report is to protect the rights of all research subjects or participants, serving as an ethical framework for medical research. There are three ethical principles: (1) respect for persons, (2) beneficence, and (3) justice (https://www.hhs.gov/ohrp/sites/default/files/the-belmont-report-508c_FINAL.pdf). The summary is presented in Table 6.4.

The approach is different from the international codes, as the Belmont Code focuses on three basic principles, particularly relevant to the ethics of research involving human subjects. These three principles are further explained in a 1979 Federal document (US Federal Register, 1979):

1. *Respect for Persons.* Respect for persons incorporates at least two ethical convictions: first, that individuals should be treated as autonomous agents, and second, that persons with diminished autonomy are entitled to protection. The principle of respect for persons thus divides into two separate moral requirements: the requirement to acknowledge autonomy and the requirement to protect those with diminished autonomy.

Table 6.4 Belmont Report

The Belmont Report – Summary
On July 12, 1974, the National Research Act (Pub. L. 93-348) was signed into law, thereby creating the National Commission for the Protection of Human Subjects of Biomedical and Behavioral Research. One of the charges to the Commission was to identify the basic ethical principles that should underlie the conduct of biomedical and behavioral research involving human subjects and to develop guidelines which should be followed to assure that such research is conducted in accordance with those principles. In carrying out the above, the Commission was directed to consider: **(i)** the boundaries between biomedical and behavioral research and the accepted and routine practice of medicine, **(ii)** the role of assessment of risk-benefit criteria in the determination of the appropriateness of research involving human subjects, **(iii)** appropriate guidelines for the selection of human subjects for participation in such research and **(iv)** the nature and definition of informed consent in various research settings.
The Belmont Report attempts to summarize the basic ethical principles identified by the Commission in the course of its deliberations. It is the outgrowth of an intensive four-day period of discussions that were held in February 1976 at the Smithsonian Institution's Belmont Conference Center supplemented by the monthly deliberations of the Commission that were held over a period of nearly four years. It is a statement of basic ethical principles and guidelines that should assist in resolving the ethical problems that surround the conduct of research with human subjects. By publishing the Report in the Federal Register, and providing reprints upon request, the Secretary intends that it may be made readily available to scientists, members of Institutional Review Boards, and Federal employees. The two-volume Appendix, containing the lengthy reports of experts and specialists who assisted the Commission in fulfilling this part of its charge, is available as DHEW Publication No. (OS) 78-0013 and No. (OS) 78-0014, for sale by the Superintendent of Documents, U.S. Government Printing Office, Washington, D.C. 20402.
Unlike most other reports of the Commission, the Belmont Report does not make specific recommendations for administrative action by the Secretary of Health, Education, and Welfare. Rather, the Commission recommended that the Belmont Report be adopted in its entirety, as a statement of the Department's policy. The Department requests public comment on this recommendation.

2. *Beneficence.* Persons are treated in an ethical manner not only by respecting their decisions and protecting them from harm, but also by making efforts to secure their well-being. Such treatment falls under the principle of beneficence. Two general rules have been formulated as complementary expressions of beneficent actions in this sense: (1) do not harm and (2) maximise possible benefits and minimise possible harms…
3. *Justice.* Who ought to receive the benefits of research and bear its burdens? This is a question of justice, in the sense of 'fairness in distribution' or 'what is deserved'. An injustice occurs when some benefit to which a person is entitled is denied without good reason or when some burden is imposed unduly…Questions of justice have long been associated with social practices such as punishment, taxation and political representation. Until recently these questions have not generally been associated with scientific research…

The Belmont Report, as explained by Sharav (2003), is the outcome of a national commission convened in reaction to the revelations of unethical experiments by American researchers.

We want to highlight two symbolic examples of these unethical experiments: first the Tuskegee syphilis study (https://www.nytimes.com/1972/07/26/archives/syphilis-victims-in-us-study-went-untreated-for-40-years-syphilis.html) and second the Willowbrook hepatitis paediatric studies (Hoop et al., 2008).

The Tuskegee syphilis study began in 1932 with about 600 African American men mostly poor and uneducated, from Tuskegee, Alabama, an area that had the highest syphilis rate in the United States at the time. There were two groups of men, 400 in the original syphilitic infected group and 200 in the control group. 'The study was conducted to determine from autopsies what the disease does to the human body… As incentives to enter the program, the men were promised free transportation to and from hospitals, free hot lunches, free medicine for any disease other than syphilis and free burial after autopsies were performed' reported the New York Times. The 400 infected patients never received deliberate treatment. Indeed, even if the study started before the availability of an efficacious treatment, that is, penicillin, once penicillin became available, the drug was denied to these men while its use probably could have helped or saved a number of them.

The Willowbrook hepatitis paediatric studies were performed at the Willowbrook State Hospital, Staten Island, New York, in the 1950s and 1960s. If parents provided consent for these studies, Hoop et al. reported that the voluntarism of their consent has been questioned because admission to the overcrowded hospital depended on the agreement to participate in the study (Hoop et al., 2008).

6.3 General ethical considerations

6.3.1 Children are not little adults

A well-known axiom in paediatrics states that children are not little adults.

Children and adolescents are more vulnerable population compared with adults.

Children and adolescents with mental disorders are doubly vulnerable (Tan and Koelch, 2008).

Stating that minors are vulnerable sounds like a tautology, however, societal pressure on adolescents seems to increase over the last decades as evidenced by some attempts to extend the cases when juveniles are or should be tried as adults for the crimes they committed. Paediatric medicine is based on a developmental approach, not only for the physical milestones but also for domains like mental maturation, competencies, or social functioning.

A 2019 paper by Bridge et al. (2019) investigated the influence of the Netflix show '13 Reasons Why' on suicide rates in American adolescents, in response to concerns expressed by mental health professionals, about adolescents being particularly sensitive to the way suicide is portrayed in the different media. '13 Reasons Why' is a series about an adolescent girl who kills herself and leaves behind a series of 13 tapes detailing the reasons why she chose to end her life. The first season received positive reviews from the critics and the public and was quite successful in terms of audience. Bridge's study was conducted across the United States by a team of researchers and clinicians at several American universities and supported by the National Institute of Mental Health (NIMH). The authors reported that '13 Reasons Why' was associated with a 28.9% increase in suicide rates among US youth ages 10–17 in the month (April 2017) following the show's release. A critical point supporting our 'plea' that minors are a more vulnerable population is that researchers did not find any significant trends in suicide rates in adults aged 18–64 years. Furthermore, they did not find any change in homicide rates supporting the idea that changes in suicide rates were influenced by the Netflix series and not by some other environmental or social factor that occurred during the same period. Of course, it is impossible to make a direct causal link between the Netflix series and the increased rate of suicide in adolescents, but it should serve as a reminder that indeed adolescents are a vulnerable population.

The ICH-E11 R1 reinforces the fundamental principle in paediatric drug development that 'children should not be enrolled in a clinical study unless necessary to achieve an important paediatric public health need'.

The concept of 'minimal risk' is difficult to define. The potential lack of apparent direct benefit for children and adolescents involved in clinical studies evidences a complex paradox of paediatric research. If the need to obtain paediatric information for medicines used in children seems a matter of consensus nowadays, the evaluation of the true benefit of participating in clinical research will instead yield varied opinions. There is no consensus of what minimal risk for paediatric patients is. Therefore discussions about risks, benefits, and burden have always to be done on a single clinical study basis.

E.3.2 Timing of studies

The ethical question about the timing of paediatric studies vis-a-vis adult development pertains obviously to new drugs or new therapeutic interventions. There is no simple answer, as many parameters have to be taken into account, making each situation rather unique. ICH E11 provides some guidance: 'During clinical development, the timing of paediatric studies will depend on the medicinal product, the type of disease being treated, safety considerations, and the efficacy and safety of alternative

Table 6.5 ICH E11 guidance on paediatric study timing based on the type of disease

Medicinal products for diseases predominantly or exclusively affecting paediatric patients
In this case the entire development program will be conducted in the paediatric population except for initial safety and tolerability data, which will usually be obtained in adults. Some products may reasonably be studied only in the paediatric population even in the initial phases, for example, when studies in adults would yield little useful information or expose them to inappropriate risk. Examples include surfactant for respiratory distress syndrome in preterm infants and therapies targeted at metabolic or genetic diseases unique to the paediatric population.
Medicinal products intended to treat serious or life-threatening diseases, occurring in both adults and paediatric patients, for which there are currently no or limited therapeutic options
The presence of a serious or life-threatening disease for which the product represents a potentially important advance in therapy suggests the need for relatively urgent and early initiation of paediatric studies. In this case, medicinal product development should begin early in the paediatric population, following assessment of initial safety data and reasonable evidence of potential benefit. Paediatric study results should be part of the marketing application database. In circumstances where this has not been possible, the lack of data should be justified in detail.
Medicinal products intended to treat other diseases and conditions
In this case, although the medicinal product will be used in paediatric patients, there is less urgency than in the previous cases, and studies would usually begin at later phases of clinical development or, if a safety concern exists, even after substantial postmarketing experience in adults. Companies should have a clear plan for paediatric studies and reasons for their timing. Testing of these medicinal products in the paediatric population would usually not begin until Phase 2 or 3. In most cases, only limited paediatric data would be available at the time of submission of the application, but more would be expected after marketing. The development of many new chemical entities is discontinued during or following Phase 1 and 2 studies in adults for lack of efficacy or an unacceptable side effect profile. Therefore very early initiation of testing in paediatric patients might needlessly expose these patients to a compound that will be of no benefit. Even for a nonserious disease, if the medicinal product represents a major therapeutic advance for the paediatric population, studies should begin early in development, and the submission of paediatric data would be expected in the application. Lack of data should be justified in detail. Thus it is important to carefully weigh benefit/risk and therapeutic need in deciding when to start paediatric studies.

treatments. Since the development of paediatric formulations can be difficult and time-consuming, it is important to consider the development of these formulations early in medicinal product development'. ICH E11 provides further guidance according to the type of disease (Table 6.5).

6.3.3 Questions to answer before involving children in clinical studies

Defining a 'ready-to-use ethical detailed checklist' before involving children in a clinical study is probably an impossible task to achieve. However, suggesting a theoretical frame to assess any paediatric study can be useful. In their book published in 1994, Grodin and Glantz (1994) proposed eight crucial questions to assess. We believe their conceptual frame remains perfectly valid, and modestly, we propose to add a ninth and a tenth point regarding input from all stakeholders, including patients/parents and recruitment strategies, especially the use of social media.

The 10 questions we, therefore, suggest are summarised in Table 6.6.

The two additional questions we propose to add to the height proposed by Grodin and Glantz in 1994 reflect the societal changes that occurred since the last century.

First, in line with the ICH E11 R1, we believe that among stakeholders from whom input should be sought, patients' representatives should be systematically considered. We strongly advocate such an approach and have devoted one chapter to this aspect 'Listening to the Patients' voice'.

Second, recruitment is always a challenge in paediatric studies, and except for studies in attention deficit hyperactivity disorder, paediatric studies are always recruiting slower than adult studies for the same condition. It is therefore of paramount

Table 6.6 Ethical assessment of paediatric studies

Ethical assessment of paediatric clinical studies
1. Is the use of children in the research study justified? Has the animal research been completed and are the results sufficiently promising to warrant studies in humans? Can the research be done in adults, thereby sparing children from involvement? Has prior research in adults produced a favourable benefit/risk ratio?
2. Is the proposed number of child subjects the fewest needed to draw meaningful conclusions? Conversely, is the study design sufficient to permit meaningful conclusions?
3. Are the proposed techniques the least intrusive possible with regard to both psychological and physical intrusion?
4. Will the research benefit the child directly? If this is not the case, are the manipulations to which the child is to be subjected minimally invasive?
5. Are the methods for obtaining assent clear and fair? Is a simplified, fair presentation made to obtain the child's assent? Is the parent present during this presentation and able to assist the investigator in interpreting to the child the demands of the studies, the anticipated benefits, and the possible risks?
6. Has every effort been made to have the parent present when the interventions occur? This often greatly reduces the burden of the research intervention upon the child.
7. Is the child with a rare disease at risk for being "over-studied"?... Such investigations may impose an excessive burden on the affected child.
8. Is money or other rewards being provided to the parent? It is appropriate to cover the expenses of the parents in enabling a child to participate in a research study. However, significant rewards for parents or for children may provide an unnecessary, inappropriate incentive for the child's participation.
9. Have patients' voices been taken into account? Among stakeholders from whom input should be sought, patients' representatives should be systematically considered.
10. Are recruitment strategies ethically sound?

Adapted from Grodin, M.A., Glantz, L.H., 1994. Children as Research Subjects. Science, Ethics and Law. Oxford University Press, Oxford, New York, Appendix A, pp. 215–217.

importance to ensure ethical paediatric recruitment. The unethical recruitment process of the Willowbrook studies, that is, linking admission to a paediatric hospital on an agreement to participate in the study illustrates well the ethical risks. We will address in more details the paediatric recruitment challenges in another chapter of this book: 'Special challenges in paediatric recruitment'.

Additionally, with the development of the use of social media as a recruitment strategy for clinical research, including paediatric research, new ethical questions may arise. We agree with Gelinas et al. (2017) that 'whether active or passive, social media recruitment should be evaluated in substantially the same way as more traditional analogue or "off-line" recruitment'. They consider that the most critical ethical considerations when dealing with social media recruitment are first respect for the privacy of social media users and second investigator transparency. They provide some concrete cases to illustrate their methodology to develop an ethical social media recruitment strategy and how to make an appropriate ethical assessment of such recruitment strategy. They suggest two checklists, one for investigators for proposing social media recruitment (that we will display in Table 6.7) and one for ethical committees and review boards to evaluate social media recruitment proposals within a US legal framework; however, their proposed checklist can be adapted to global studies and different legal frames.

The authors did not look at paediatric specificities, however, citing the success of social media recruitment in paediatric cancer studies. While parents or caregivers and adolescents often agree about research decisions, we believe that social media recruitment may create potentially some more complex situations than with tradition recruitment campaigns; adolescents generally using more than their parents social media might be the first aware of a potential study and might even be the ones first to contact research teams.

Paediatric patients due to their inherent immaturity and vulnerability do not have the legal right to consent their participation in clinical research. Ultimately, parental involvement is required, framing the concept of parental permission and child assent. Children and adolescents suffering from mental disorders may experience additional difficulties in deciding about their participation in clinical research. Researches on adolescent assent have emphasised the fact that the assent process is highly contextualised nature and, therefore, social media recruitment has the potential to induce more debates between parents, adolescents, and researchers.

Therefore we would suggest a seventh point (Table 6.8) on how to handle direct contacts from adolescents or minors in general and how to potentially handle discordance between adolescents and parents about participation in clinical research.

6.3.4 Feasibility

We will not discuss feasibility in detail in this chapter, as this Klaudius Siegfried does this in the following chapter 'Running clinical trials'. However, as we mentioned in other parts of this book, poor design may lead to recruitment difficulties, to early termination of a study before its completion, well-conducted and credible feasibility has an essential ethical role as well in helping to ensure that children and adolescents will not be exposed to clinical study procedures for nothing.

Table 6.7 Checklist for proposing social media recruitment

Investigator checklist for proposing social media recruitment (Gelinas et al., 2017)

Investigators proposing to recruit via social media are advised to take the following steps:
1. Provide the IRB with a statement describing the proposed social media recruitment techniques, including the following:
   – A list of the sites to be used.
   – A description of whether recruitment will be passive and/or active.
   – If utilising active recruitment, a description of how potential participants will be identified and approached, and their privacy maintained.
2. Ensure that the social media recruitment strategy complies with applicable federal and state laws
3. Provide the IRB with a statement certifying compliance (or lack of noncompliance) with the policies and terms of use of relevant websites, OR if proposed techniques **conflict** with relevant website policies and terms of use:
   – Seek an exception from the website to its terms of use; provide the IRB with written documentation of the exception, if granted.
   – Depending on IRB policy, in compelling circumstances make the case that the recruitment strategy should be allowed to proceed in the absence of an exception from the site.
4. Ensure that the proposed recruitment strategy respects all relevant ethical norms, including the following:
   – Proposed recruitment does not involve deception or fabrication of online identities.
   – Trials are accurately represented in recruitment overtures.
   – Proposed recruitment does not involve members of research team 'lurking' or 'creeping' social media sites in ways members are unaware of.
   – Recruitment will not involve advancements or contact that could embarrass or stigmatise potential participants.
5. If the research team intends to recruit from the online networks of current or potential study participants:
   – Provide the IRB with a statement explaining this approach and describing plans to obtain consent and documentation of consent from participants before approaching members of their online networks or to invite the individual themselves to approach members of their network on the research team's behalf.
6. Consider whether a formal communication plan is needed for managing social media activities among enrolled participants, including the following:
   – steps to educate participants about the importance of blinding and how certain communications can jeopardise the scientific validity of a study (e.g. a section in the orientation or consent form)
   – triggers for intervention from the research team (e.g. misinformation or speculation among participants on social media that could lead to unblinding)
   – interventions from the research team (e.g. corrections of misinformation or reminders about importance of blinding on social media)

E.3.4.1 Submission to Institutional Review Board/Independent Ethics Committee (IRB/IEC)

The roles and responsibilities of Independent Ethics Committees (IECs)/Institutional Review Boards (IRBs) are not detailed in ICH E11 but in ICH E6 (https://www.ich.org/fileadmin/Public_Web_Site/ICH_Products/Guidelines/Efficacy/E6/E6_R1_Guideline.pdf).

Table 6.8 Paediatric social media addendum

Investigator checklist for proposing social media recruitment – Paediatric addendum

7. Ensure a working process is put in place to handle paediatric specificities
  – Ensure a specific process is operational in case of minors, mainly adolescents, contact the research teams directly
  – Ensure an adequate process is in place to facilitate a constructive discussion between parents, adolescents and researchers for an ethical decision-making process

Independent Ethics Committees and Institutional Review Boards have a crucial role in the protection of study participants. When reviewing paediatric clinical trial protocols, IEC/IRB representatives should have expertise within paediatric clinical, scientific, and ethical aspects. ICH E11 suggests consulting experts knowledgeable in psychosocial issues as well. Continuous dialogue between competent authorities, IRBs/ECs, patients and parents' associations, and industry representatives on paediatric development programmes is considered needed and beneficial for all parties concerned. In this respect, it can be useful when submitting a clinical study protocol to an IEC/IRB to submit an additional cover letter detailing the current scientific knowledge and the ethical considerations in more details than what is usually written in a protocol; in our experience, this has been a useful way to engage a constructive dialogue.

6.3.4.2 Consent, assent, and competence

The voluntary participation of human subjects and transparent and accurate information about the research are absolutely essential. The Belmont report of 1979 outlines three basic ethical principles for the protection of subjects, that is, respect for persons, beneficence, and justice. Research in such a vulnerable population of mentally ill minors introduces more complexity, a doubly vulnerable population (Tan and Koelch, 2008). Not only parental permission or parental consent and child assent have to be sought, but also all the psychopathological representations and emotional conflicts inherent of mental disorders have not to be forgotten when designing and implementing a clinical study.

The parental informed consent is following a process close to an adult informed consent. It should provide precise and understandable study information to the parents and caregivers, set up clear and fair expectations, and take into account specific family needs. Parents should understand the difference between research and therapy and understand the trial procedures and the investigator, and the study team should thoroughly explain the alternative therapeutic strategy.

The child assent process means further challenges. It is defined as a child's affirmative agreement to participate in research, and further clarification is given that 'mere failure to object should not, absent affirmative agreement, be construed as assent'. (Shaddy and Denne, 2010). The American Academy of Pediatrics recommends that active agreement by a minor (not qualified to give consent) to participate in a research study generally applies to children who have reached an intellectual age of at least 7 years. More recently, it was suggested that assent is generally applicable to developmentally normal children between 8 and 14 years of age (Shaddy and Denne, 2010). The assent should provide understandable study information and expectations. At the age of 14 years, it is usually considered that adolescents have reached adult level information.

ICH E11 introduces two additional points to the original text:

- The fact that throughout a clinical study, it may be necessary to reassess the assent of a child or an adolescent in recognition of their advancing age, evolving maturity, and competency. This applies primarily to long-term studies, like some of the 2-year safety studies that have been requested by the EMA; an obvious example is clinical studies where children become adolescents.
- The need to follow regulations related to confidentiality and privacy of paediatric patients; the increased use of social media illustrates this critical "new" requirement.

Table 6.9 summarises the ICH E11 and ICH E11 (R1) position about consent and assent.

Table 6.9 Consent and assent – ICH E11

ICH E11
As a rule, a paediatric subject is legally unable to provide informed consent. Therefore paediatric study participants are dependent on their parent(s)/legal guardian to assume responsibility for their participation in clinical studies. Fully informed consent should be obtained from the legal guardian in accordance with regional laws or regulations. All participants should be informed to the fullest extent possible about the study in language and terms they are able to understand. Where appropriate, participants should assent to enrol in a study (age of assent to be determined by IRB's/IEC's or be consistent with local legal requirements). Participants of appropriate intellectual maturity should personally sign and date either a separately designed, written assent form or the written informed consent. In all cases, participants should be made aware of their rights to decline to participate or to withdraw from the study at any time. Attention should be paid to signs of undue distress in patients who are unable to clearly articulate their distress. Although a participant's wish to withdraw from a study must be respected, there may be circumstances in therapeutic studies for serious or life-threatening diseases in which, in the opinion of the investigator and parent(s)/legal guardian, the welfare of a paediatric patient would be jeopardised by his or her failing to participate in the study. In this situation, continued parental (legal guardian) consent should be sufficient to allow participation in the study. Emancipated or mature minors (defined by local laws) may be capable of giving autonomous consent. Information that can be obtained in a less vulnerable, consenting population should not be obtained in a more vulnerable population or one in which the patients are unable to provide individual consent. Studies in handicapped or institutionalised paediatric populations should be limited to diseases or conditions found principally or exclusively in these populations, or situations in which the disease or condition in these paediatric patients would be expected to alter the disposition or pharmacodynamic effects of a medicinal product.

Continued

Table 6.9 Continued

> ICH E11 (R1)
> The general principles of ethical considerations for parental (legal guardian) consent/permission and child assent are outlined in ICH E11 (2000) Section 2.6.3 and continue to apply. Information regarding participation in the clinical study and the process of parental (legal guardian) consent/permission and child assent must be clearly provided to the parent (legal guardian) and as appropriate to the child participant, at the time of enrollment. When obtaining child assent, relevant elements of informed consent should be provided that are appropriate to the child's capability to understand. Refusal to assent or withdrawal of assent by a child should be respected.
> Over the course of a clinical study, it may be necessary to reassess the assent of a child in recognition of their advancing age, evolving maturity and competency, especially for long-term studies or studies that may require sample retention. During clinical studies there is a requirement for obtaining adequate informed consent for continued participation from paediatric participants once a child reaches the age of legal consent. Local regulations related to confidentiality and privacy of paediatric participants must be followed.

6.3.5 Cultural differences

Child and adolescent psychiatry is a rather young discipline, not recognised nor established as a medical speciality worldwide, evidencing noticeable differences in cultural approaches. We believe the ethical aspects of research are universal. The need to understand cultural differences, regardless of the specificity of psychiatry, should still result in aligning the ethical requirements. The ICH E11 revision adds: 'Pediatric drug development programs are increasingly multiregional, and these programs face specific challenges due to regional differences in pediatric regulatory requirements, operational practicalities, standards of care, and cultural expectations'. These differences will be discussed in the chapter focusing on 'Running clinical trials'.

6.3.6 Potential conflict of interest

Last but not least, it is crucial to assess any potential risk of conflict of interest. There has a growing concern vis-à-vis commercially funded research, as potential financial conflicts of interest from investigators conducting clinical trials may compromise the well-being of research subjects. Financial conflicts of interest may undermine trust in clinical research. We believe that policies governing conflicts of interest in clinical trials should be strict and transparent; control institutions have an essential role to play.

ICH E11 (R1) adds that the transparency of paediatric clinical research includes the registration of clinical trials on publicly accessible and recognised databases and the public availability of clinical trial results, and we will discuss the latter in a specific chapter of this book.

6.4 Conclusion

Over the last two decades, the growing concern regarding the off-label use of medicines in children and their limited access to new or innovative medications has led to paediatric regulations recognising that such a situation is unethical.

However, the solution to increasing psychopharmacological research is not widely understood and not necessarily perceived as an ethical answer. However, would the ethical answer remain prescribing drugs to children and adolescents without any paediatric information, meaning accepting lower standards for paediatric patients compared with the adult population? Therefore our book supports the need to obtain paediatric information, including via clinical studies in children and adolescents. We do not forget that medical research has a horrible dark history with the rights of human beings being repetitively violated by physicians and researchers.

The discussion of ethical aspects of paediatric research is a central point, and we suggest to summarise each study/programme assessment by using the following three primary considerations:

- Is the research, including its operational aspects, scientifically justified and ethical?
- Have the issues of consent and competence been addressed?
- Has the potential conflict of interest been assessed?

We hope that we have been able to modestly contribute to the understanding of the challenges of ensuring highest paediatric ethical standards.

References

Bridge, J.A., Greenhouse, J.B., Ruch, D., Stevens, J., Ackerman, J., Sheftall, A.H., Horowitz, L.M., Kelleher, K.J., Campo, J.V., 2019. Association between the release of Netflix's 13 reasons why and suicide rates in the United States: an interrupted times series analysis. J. Am. Acad. Child Adolesc. Psychiatry. https://doi.org/10.1016/j.jaac.2019.04.020.
Gelinas, L., Pierce, R., Winkler, S., Cohen, I.G., Lynch, H.F., Bierer, B.E., 2017. Using social media as a research recruitment tool: ethical issues and recommendations. Am. J. Bioeth. 17 (3), 3–14.
Ghooi, R.B., 2011. The Nuremberg Code – a critique. Perspect. Clin. Res. 2 (2), 72–76.
Grodin, M.A., Glantz, L.H., 1994. Children as Research Subjects. Science, Ethics and Law. Oxford University Press, Oxford, New York.
Hoop, J.G., Smyth, A.C., Roberts, L.W., 2008. Ethical issues in psychiatric research on children and adolescents. Child Adolesc. Psychiatr. Clin. N. Am. 17 (1), 127–148.
JAMA, 1964. WMA's declaration of Helsinki serves as guide to physicians. JAMA 189 (13), 33–34. https://doi.org/10.1001/jama.1964.03070130073046.
LaFleur, W.R., Böhme, G., Shimazono, S. (Eds.), 2007. Dark Medicine: Rationalizing Unethical Medical Research. Project Muse. Indiana University Press.
Moreno, J.D., Schmidt, U., Joffe, S., 2017. The Nuremberg code 70 years later. JAMA 318 (9), 795–796. https://doi.org/10.1001/jama.2017.10265.
Parsa-Parsi, R.W., 2017. The revised declaration of Geneva: a modern-day physician's pledge. JAMA 318 (20), 1971–1972.

Shaddy, R.E., Denne, S.C., 2010. Clinical report – guidelines for the ethical conduct of studies to evaluate drugs in pediatric populations. Pediatrics 125 (4), 850–860.
Sharav, V.H., 2003. Children in clinical research: A conflict of moral values. Am. J. Bioeth. 3 (1). InFocus.
Tan, J.O., Koelch, M., 2008. The ethics of psycho-pharmacological research in legal minors. Child Adolesc. Psychiatry Ment. Health 2 (1), 39.
US Federal Register, 1979. US Federal Register/Vol. 44, No. 76/Wednesday, April 18, 1979/ Notices Part IV – Department of Health, Education, and Welfare – Office of the Secretary – Protection of Human Subjects; Notice of Report for Public Comment.

Further reading

https://history.nih.gov/research/downloads/nuremberg.pdf.
https://sites.jamanetwork.com/research-ethics/index.html.
https://www.hhs.gov/ohrp/sites/default/files/the-belmont-report-508c_FINAL.pdf.
https://www.ich.org/fileadmin/Public_Web_Site/ICH_Products/Guidelines/Efficacy/E6/E6_R1_Guideline.pdf.
https://www.nytimes.com/1972/07/26/archives/syphilis-victims-in-us-study-went-untreated-for-40-years-syphilis.html.

Study design and methodology

Philippe Auby
Otsuka Pharmaceutical Development & Commercialisation Europe, Frankfurt am Main, Germany

7.1 Introduction

Paediatric development is fortunately nowadays strictly controlled by numerous regulations. Still, regulations cannot suffice. It is of paramount importance to ensure that paediatric development is scientifically and ethically sound. Study design and methodology are indeed among the key factors to ensure a successful and meaningful conclusive outcome. Not completing paediatric trials because of poor design should not be accepted. We are not going to solve the issues of paediatric study design and methodology in this chapter, but we will emphasise the fundamental principles as clearly defined by the ICH E11 and use the paediatric studies with antidepressants in major depressive disorders as an illustration of the challenges, letting the issue of indiscriminative studies to be explored in details by Klaudius Siegfried in a following chapter. Children are a vulnerable population, depending on adults for protection including when considering their participation in a clinical trial.

7.2 ICE 11, the reference for paediatric research

In July 2000 the ICH E11 was approved by the ICH Steering Committee and recommended for adoption to the three ICH regulatory bodies, the United States, EU, and Japan (https://www.ich.org/home.html). The objectives of this new ICH guidance were to 'encourage and facilitate timely paediatric medicinal product development internationally' by providing 'an outline of critical issues in paediatric drug development and approaches to the safe, efficient, and ethical study of medicinal products in the paediatric population' focusing on the following topics:

1. considerations when initiating a paediatric programme for a medicinal product
2. timing of initiation of paediatric studies during medicinal product development
3. types of studies (pharmacokinetic, pharmacokinetic/pharmacodynamic (PK/PD), efficacy, and safety)
4. age categories
5. ethics of paediatric clinical investigation

The ICH E11 clearly defines the essential points to consider for any paediatric medicinal development (Table 7.1).
The ICH E11 established a clear frame and a real ambition that all regulations translate in their expectations for paediatric drug development. Triggered by these

Table 7.1 ICH E11

ICH E11: Issues when initiating a paediatric medicinal product development programme
• The prevalence of the condition to be treated in the paediatric population • The seriousness of the condition to be treated • The availability and suitability of alternative treatments for the condition in the paediatric population, including the efficacy and the adverse event profile (including any unique paediatric safety issues) of those treatments • Whether the medicinal product is novel or one of a class of compounds with known properties • Whether there are unique paediatric indications for the medicinal product • The need for the development of paediatric-specific endpoints • The age ranges of paediatric patients likely to be treated with the medicinal product • Unique paediatric (developmental) safety concerns with the medicinal product, including any nonclinical safety issues • Potential need for paediatric formulation development Of these factors the most important is the presence of a serious or life-threatening disease for which the medicinal product represents a potentially important advance in therapy. This situation suggests relatively urgent and early initiation of paediatric studies

regulations, paediatric drug development has evolved rather fast over the last two decades, and understanding these changes, 15 years after the ICH E11 was released, in 2017, the ICH published the addendum (R1). This addendum signals that a full revision is not deemed necessary; therefore it does not alter the scope of the original guideline but complements it and provides new perspectives on paediatric drug development. Interestingly, this addendum is taking into account a very complex aspect of paediatric development, that is, the fact that differences do exist between the ways paediatric development is considered across the different regions. The ICH aims to 'reduce the likelihood that substantial differences will exist among regions for the acceptance of data generated in paediatric global drug development programs'. Specifically, Section 3 addresses this challenging question on the commonality of the scientific approach across different regions.

If the US paediatric regulation paved the way of paediatric drug development, the EU paediatric regulation offered a second frame that formally enables dialogues between the different regions to develop a more global approach to bring better medicines for children worldwide. The recent Swiss paediatric regulation supports global paediatric drug development by bridging with the existing US and EU regulations. In practice, paediatric drug development and paediatric studies are more and more conducted in numerous countries and different parts of the world, where 'differences in paediatric regulatory requirements, operational practicalities, standards of care, and cultural expectations' create significant challenges. To address such differences the ICH E11 (R1) suggests considering the following questions that are summarised in Table 7.2 with reference to the different sections of the document.

Additionally the ICH E11 (R1) mentions that among stakeholders from whom input should be sought, patients' representatives should be considered. We believe this is an

Study design and methodology

Table 7.2 ICH E11 (R1)

ICH E11 (R1): Commonality of scientific approach for paediatric drug development programmes
• What is the medical need in one or more paediatric populations that the drug could address? • Who are the appropriate paediatric populations or subgroups that could be considered? (See Section 4) • What are the key issues in the drug development programme that need to be addressed based on the intended paediatric use of the drug? • Based on the existing knowledge, including developmental physiology, disease pathophysiology, nonclinical data, data in adult or paediatric populations, or data from related compounds, what are the knowledge gaps that should be addressed to establish the safe and effective use of the drug? (See Section 5.1) • What specific nonclinical studies could be considered? • What clinical studies and/or methodological approaches could be considered? (See Section 5) • What paediatric-specific clinical study design elements could be considered? (See Section 5) • What practical and operational issues should be considered? (See Sections 4 and 6) • Are there different formulations/dosage forms or delivery devices that will be needed for specific paediatric subgroups, both to facilitate an optimal dose-finding strategy, and for the treatment of paediatric patients in different subgroups? (See Section 7) A common scientific approach should consider input from stakeholders (e.g. clinicians, patients, and experts from academia) and should be based on scientific advances and up-to-date knowledge

important shift that developers need to consider systematically, and we advocate such an approach, to listen to the patients' voices (cf. Listening to the Patients' Voice chapter).

Other additions to the ICH E11 are Section 6 on practicalities in the design and execution of paediatric clinical studies and Section 5 on approaches to optimise paediatric drug development considering paediatric extrapolation and introducing modelling and simulation. We are not going to discuss in this chapter extrapolation, modelling, and simulation, and we have mentioned it in the historical perspective chapter. However, we would like to use this topic to emphasise the fact that paediatric drug development is an evolving field. For instance, in Europe, the PDCO has recently repetitively accepted study extrapolation instead of clinical studies along with the evidence from the literature to support the maintenance of antipsychotic effect of new pharmacological agents in adolescents with schizophrenia.

Section 7 supplements ICH E11 on paediatric formulations, a major and often underestimated paediatric drug development topic. This aspect will not be developed in this book as we would instead recommend our readers to read *Pediatric Formulations: A Roadmap* the excellent book by Daniel Bar-Shalom and Klaus Rose that provides a thorough overview of the importance of age-appropriate paediatric formulations, defining their challenges; drawing an overview of the existing technologies; and suggesting a roadmap to better, innovative formulations, in particular for oral administration (Bar-Shalom and Rose, 2014).

Section 4 on age classification and paediatric subgroups further discuss the somewhat arbitrary (and clearly presented as only one possible classification in the ICH E11) chronological classification. Indeed, for child and adolescent psychopharmacology, the 'Children' subgroup, that is, 2–11 years of age, is heterogeneous, and the rule of paediatric development is to only consider, depending on the study disorder, part of this subgroup for pharmacological intervention. On the other end of the paediatric spectrum, the 'Adolescent' subgroup may offer the opportunity to consider including adolescents in adult studies for certain conditions and certain studies. The FDA and the EMA have already supported this approach. The ICH E11 (R1) is going even further in questioning the age boundaries: 'Depending on factors such as the condition, the treatment, and the study design, it may be justifiable to include paediatric subpopulations in adult studies (see Section 6) or adult subpopulations in paediatric studies'.

7.3 Evolving nature of study design and methodology

Triggered first by the United States and then the EU regulations, the number of paediatric studies has increased over the last years. Not all of these studies are part of a regulatory frame showing also that the shift from protecting children from studies to protecting children by conducting studies that will enhance the paediatric knowledge is occurring. In 2015 Persico et al. published an important article about 'Unmet needs in paediatric psychopharmacology: Present scenario and future perspectives' (Persico et al., 2015) demonstrating the striking lack of pharmacological therapeutic options available in child and adolescent psychiatry. A few years later, their statement remains valid despite new agents being approved. Fig. 7.1 as discussed later is an update and

Table 2 Psychotropic medications approved in Europe for use in children and adolescents. 2015

Medication	Indication	Age for prescription
Aripiprazole	Schizophrenia	≥ 15 years
	Bipolar disorder, manic or mixed episodes	≥ 13 years
Amphetamines (incl. Lisdexamphetamine)	Attention-Deficit Hyperactivity Disorder[a]	≥ 6 years
Atomoxetine	Attention-Deficit Hyperactivity Disorder	≥ 6 years
Fluoxetine	Major depressive episode	≥ 8 years
Fluvoxamine	Obsessive-compulsive disorder	≥ 8 years
Methylphenidate	Attention-Deficit hyperactivity Disorder	≥ 6 years
Risperidone	Aggression[b]	≥ 5 years
Sertraline	Obsessive-compulsive disorder	≥ 6 years
Ziprasidone	Bipolar disorder, manic or mixed episode[c]	≥ 10 years

[a]Approved only in some European countries for children and adolescents with ADHD.
[b]Approved only in some European countries for children and adolescents with conduct disorder, in the presence of sub-average intellectual functioning or intellectual disability and when all non-pharmacological strategies have been found insufficient.
[c]Approved only in some European countries based on one randomized controlled trial (Findling et al., 2013), found by the US Food and Drug Administration to have quality assurance issues, requiring the sponsor to repeat the trial.

			Since 2015
Paliperidone	Schizophrenia	≥ 15 years	
Melatonin	Insomnia in ASD	≥ 2 years	
Guanfacine	ADHD	≥ 6 years	

Fig. 7.1 Psychotropic medications currently approved in Europe for use in children and adolescents.

adaptation of their article's Table 7.2 presenting all psychotropic medications currently approved in Europe for use in children and adolescents.

Only one selective serotonin uptake inhibitor (SSRI), fluoxetine, is approved in EU for the treatment of paediatric MDD. In the United States, further to fluoxetine, escitalopram is approved for adolescents only. The lack of approved antidepressant is not due to the lack of clinical studies. The US paediatric regulation triggered a significant number of paediatric efficacy studies in children and adolescents with MDD. Unfortunately, contrary to what was reported in adults, paediatric studies were mainly negative or inconclusive, the variability of placebo response rates being the most critical differentiator between positive and negative studies. This issue of indiscriminate paediatric studies is thoroughly discussed in the third chapter focusing on study design and methodology (K. Siegfried, Indiscriminant efficacy results and the placebo issue).

Fig. 7.2 summarises the outcomes of paediatric efficacy MDD studies with all antidepressants (except tricyclics) and is adapted from the FDA 2003 reports based on two metaanalyses of 20 placebo-controlled studies involving approximately 4400 patients issued when, prompted by reports of suicidality associated with SSRIs, the efficacy and safety of these drugs in paediatric MDD were reviewed by the FDA. Following this review the FDA issued a 'black box' warning on the use of antidepressants in paediatric patients in 2014. In December 2004 the EMEA, through the Committee for

Summary of Efficacy Results for Short-Term Placebo-Controlled Paediatric Studies in MDD – 2003 (FDA)			
Drug Program/Study Number	**Age Range**	**Outcome[1] (Drug vs Placebo)**	
Paroxetine/329	12-18	Negative[2]	1.Positive (p≤0.05); Negative (p>0.10); Trend (0.05<p≤0.10)
Paroxetine/377	13-18	Negative	
Paroxetine/701	7-17	Negative	2.Keller, et al, 2001; positive on most secondary endpoints
Fluoxetine/HCJE	8-17	Positive	
Fluoxetine/X065	8-17	Positive	3.Wagner, et al, 2003; positive on pooling of 2 studies
Sertraline/A050-1001	6-17	Trend	
Sertraline/A050-1017	6-17	Negative[3]	
Venlafaxine/382	7-17	Negative	2 and 3 are further discussed in the last chapter of the book (about publications)
Venlafaxine/394	7-17	Negative	
Citalopram/CIT-MD-18	7-17	Positive	
Citalopram/94404	13-18	Negative	
Nefazodone/CN104-141	12-18	Trend	
Nefazodone/CN104-187	7-17	Negative	
Mirtazapine/003-004/Study 1	7-17	Negative	
Mirtazapine/003-004/Study 2	7-17	Negative	
Paediatric Studies in MDD – 2003 – to date			
Escitalopram 2 studies	12-18	Positive / Trend	
Duloxetine 2 studies	7-17	Negative	
Selegiline 1 study	12-17	Negative	
Desvenlafaxine 2 studies	7-18	Negative	

Fig. 7.2 Summary of efficacy for paediatric MDD studies.

Medicinal Products for Human Use (CHMP), also advised against using these medications in children and adolescents based on the reports of increased risk of suicide attempts and suicidal thoughts in clinical studies and, in April 2005, recommended that they should only be used for their approved indications (to date, only fluoxetine for paediatric MDD).

Tricyclic antidepressants seem to show some marginal evidence of efficacy in adolescents only (not in younger patients) with MDD, however, not strongly supporting their use in adolescents, as their efficacy seems to be moderate at best and their safety and tolerability profile far from being benign making their benefit/risk rather negative (Hazell et al., 1995). The authors even suggested that research should be directed towards the evaluation of the newer antidepressants and nondrug therapeutic interventions.

When SSRIs were introduced, there was much interest among the community of child and adolescent psychiatrists for these new safer antidepressants. Moreover, their clinical experience seemed to confirm their expectations that SSRIs were often beneficial when prescribed wisely, to paediatric patients with MDD. Therefore the disconnection and even the discrepancy between the clinical experience and the results of the clinical studies with SSRIs in paediatric MDD were not only frustrating but also questioning the methodology of these trials. The reasons why many of the efficacy studies failed are quite diverse, multiple, and somewhat still putative, from potential age-related differences in pharmacokinetics and pharmacodynamics and methodological flaws (with regard to patient recruitment, study design, inclusion and exclusion criteria, lack of dose-finding studies, site selection, or correlation between greater placebo response and high number of study sites) to high placebo response in paediatric depression. We want to refer two interesting articles one from Emslie et al. in (2005) and one from Bridge et al. (2009). However, what we can learn from the methodological questions is that in the field of child and adolescent psychopharmacology, probably more than in the adult field, study design and methodology should never be a replication of a past successful experience. Clearly, it is of paramount importance to learn from different sources of information (as stated in the ICH E11 R), and surprisingly, little has been published on how researchers use the available information. A survey published in 2005 by Cooper et al. showed surprising results among researchers cited in the Cochrane in the 2002 and 2003 updated 1996 reviews; actually, even the results should be interpreted cautiously, they reported that the proportion of study investigators using systematic reviews including Cochrane's was quite limited.

Two new paediatric MDD programmes are currently ongoing, one with esketamine in adolescents with MDD with imminent risk for suicide (MDSI) and vortioxetine in children and adolescents from 7 years of age with MDD (Auby, 2018). These two programmes are exciting in the sense that they are proposing new venues, looking at a paediatric population of patients de facto excluded from clinical trials with esketamine or conducting separate studies in children and adolescents with vortioxetine as the therapeutic response may be different between children and adolescents. These two paediatric developments illustrate that the need to explore innovative study designs should be explored, like the sequential parallel comparison design (SPCD) proposed by M. Fava. The SPCD consists of two phases of equal duration, with 6 weeks representing a common choice. In recent years, SPCD trials have utilised the following twophase format: Unequal randomization is applied between active drug and placebo, with more subjects allocated to placebo; then, at the end of the first phase, placebo nonresponders are rerandomised usually with equal allocation to placebo or active drug. This design enables to reduce the number of arms and limit the sample size, therefore, the number of sites and the probability and expectation of receiving placebo (Fava et al., 2003). There are also lessons to be learned from nonindustry-sponsored studies and real-life data; the best example is the work performed by I. Goodyer et al. in Cambridge, first with the 'Adolescent Depression Antidepressant and Psychotherapy Trial (ADAPT)', in adolescents aged 11–17 years with MDD published in 2007 (Goodyer et al., 2007), and second the 'Cognitive–behavioural therapy and short-term psychoanalytic psychotherapy versus brief psychosocial intervention in adolescents with unipolar major depression (IMPACT)' published in 2017 (Goodyer et al., 2017). The ADAPT trial suggests that the combination of CBT and SSRI only has a modest advantage over an SSRI alone in treating depression in adolescents and therefore that monotherapy with an SSRI is a reasonable treatment option for moderate to severe depression in adolescents, particularly if access to CBT is delayed.

7.4 Fundamental paediatric principles of study design and methodology

As children are not little adults, paediatric studies are not simple cosmetic adaptations of adult protocols. Taking such a path would probably be the recipe for failure. Poor design may lead to recruitment difficulties and at worse ending a clinical study before its completion. Further to inappropriate use of research resources and a missed scientific opportunity, exposing children to clinical studies that discontinue prematurely raise serious ethical concerns. We will develop more this question in the 'Special Challenges in Paediatric Recruitment' chapter. Still, this issue of premature discontinuation of clinical trials remains a concern. In a paper published in 2016, N. Pica and F. Bourgeois reported that for five paediatric trials, one was early discontinued. They conducted a retrospective, cross-sectional study of all paediatric randomised clinical trials registered in https://clinicaltrials.gov from 2008 to 2010, collecting data from the registry and associated publications until 1 September 2015. They identified 559 paediatric randomised clinical trials; among these 559 studies, 104 (19%) were discontinued early. Studies were less likely to be discontinued if they were sponsored by the pharmaceutical industry compared with academic institutions (odds ratio (OR) 0.46, 95% confidence interval (CI) 0.27–0.77). Poor recruitment and problems with the operational aspects of the studies were among the most commonly reported reasons for study discontinuation. Despite methodological limitations, such reported high discontinuation rate is ethically concerning as it means that approximately 8369 children were 'exposed' to 'medical testing' for no valid reason. The authors concluded: 'Although policies and initiatives have been implemented to increase the number of pediatric trials and improve the standards of trial reporting overall, further action is needed to ensure that the participation of all children in clinical trials contributes to our scientific knowledge'.

It would be essential to perform further cross-sectional studies of paediatric randomised clinical trials to understand the evolution of the percentage of early discontinued studies.

7.5 Discussion: practical points to consider when designing a paediatric study

The crucial point is 'knowledge' and knowing what as a researcher (s) you/we know and what you/we do not know. The ICH E11 (R1) states elegantly: 'A common scientific approach should consider input from stakeholders (e.g. clinicians, patients, experts from academia) and should be based on scientific advances and up-to-date knowledge.' Except for ADHD, experience has repetitively shown that paediatric studies in child and adolescent psychopharmacology are harder to perform than adult ones.

We are not going to give a kind of paediatric checklist but would like to share some fundamental points to consider when writing a paediatric protocol.

7.5.1 Study population

One striking difference between adult and paediatric patients is that in the field of child and adolescent psychiatry, comorbidity is the rule rather than the exception (Caron and Rutter, 1991): clinical and epidemiological investigations have revealed that 40%–70% of depressed children and adolescents have comorbid psychiatric disorders and that at least 20%–50% have two or more comorbid diagnoses. Therefore it is crucial to ensure that all investigators are enrolling the same patients as clinical practices do vary between researchers and not only between country locations. Making a proper and reliable diagnosis is not easy and should always be performed by an experienced and adequately trained clinician. Therefore especially for large clinical studies, we would recommend using a two-step diagnosis process. First the diagnosis of the primary studied disorder should be clinical, based on international classifications, as the DSM-5 criteria and made by an adequately trained clinician with experience with the study population (e.g. but not restricted to, by a child and adolescent psychiatrist). The diagnosis should then be confirmed by utilising a semistructured interview, the Kiddie Schedule for Affective Disorders and Schizophrenia for School-aged Children, Present and Lifetime Version (K-SADS-PL – DSM-5; Kaufman et al., 2016), at the time of screening, administered by an adequately trained clinician. The K-SADS-PL DSM-5 is a semistructured diagnostic interview designed to assess current and past psychiatric disorders in children and adolescents (aged 6–18 years) according to DSM-5 criteria.

This is an important point to consider as if the studied population does not reflect the reality of the patients who will be treated in real life, generalisability of the study results is far from guaranteed.

Just like children are not small adults, paediatric protocols are not a simple adaptation of adult studies. We would recommend to researchers in pharmaceutical companies to start with 'fresh eyes' and develop a specific paediatric template that would avoid as much as possible significant mistakes that could lead to rejection by ethics committees or significant operational difficulties leading to recruitment issues and potentially early discontinuation of the trial.

Initiatives like TransCelerate are ongoing to develop Common Protocol Template (CPT) a harmonised and streamlined approach to the format and content of clinical trial protocols. It aims to ease interpretation by the study sites and global regulatory authorities while enabling downstream automation of many clinical processes and aligning to industry data standards. At present, there is no CPT in the field of child and adolescent psychopharmacology.

7.5.2 Clinical assessments

Particular attention should be given to assessment tools, and scales appropriate for children (depending on age group) have to be used. Basically, two approaches have been followed. One way is to develop specific paediatric scales, for instance, the Children Depression Rating Scale-Revised (CDRS-R) to assess depressive symptoms. This 17-item scale based on a semistructured interview with the child (or an adult informant) is designed and validated for children aged 6–12 years; it is also used for adolescents (Poznanski and Mokros, 1996). The CDRS-R is considered as the 'gold standard' for the measure of treatment outcome in paediatric MDD and requires specific training. The other approach when appropriate was to validate adult scales in the paediatric population like what was done for the Young Mania Rating Scale (Y-MRS) as explained by Youngstrom et al. (2005). This 11-item scale is based on child/adolescent self-reporting and clinician observation. The Y-MRS is considered the 'gold standard' for the measure of treatment outcome in paediatric mania and also requires specific training.

For the safety assessments, we would like to refer the readers to the 'Specificities of Safety Management in Paediatric Psychopharmacological Research' chapter, however, emphasising the need to include long-term safety studies to assess effects on physical and cognitive development and maturation.

For parents and healthcare professionals, it does suffice to get positive results of a paediatric study showing a significant improvement over placebo or even some advantages over current therapeutic options; it is of equal importance to get paediatric patient-reported outcomes (PROs) and a clear signal that paediatric patients are functioning, simply able to go back to school, to interact with peers, and to function within their family. Regulators have supported this thought process, and PRO data are increasingly used to support paediatric labelling claims. A task force associated with the International Society for Pharmacoeconomics and Outcomes Research (ISPOR) recommended good practices for paediatric PRO research that is conducted to inform regulatory decision-making and support claims (Matza et al., 2013). They suggested the five following good research practices (Table 7.3).

Table 7.3 IPSOR five paediatric good research practices

	Comments and recommendations
1. Consider developmental differences and determine age-based criteria for PRO administration	– Four age groups are discussed. These age groups should be used as a starting point when making decisions. It is not possible to provide age cutoffs that will fit every situation. Specific age cutoffs should be determined individually for each PRO instrument and tested with cognitive interviews in each new target population – Less than 5 years old: No clear evidence of reliability or validity of child-report measures – 5–7 years old: Child-report is possible, but reliability and validity are often questionable – 8–11 years old: Reliability and validity of child-report improves – 12–18 years old: Self-report is preferred
2. Establish content validity of paediatric PRO instruments	– Children and adolescents can be effective content experts – In most cases, children should be included in qualitative research performed to establish content validity of paediatric PROs – Cognitive interviews should be conducted with the intended respondent. Children should be interviewed for child-report instruments, and parents should be interviewed for parent-report instruments – Content validity should be demonstrated within narrow age groupings
3. Determine whether an informant-reported outcome instrument is necessary	– Informant-reported outcomes include both proxy and observational measures – When children in the target age range are capable of completing a PRO instrument independently, a child-reported measure should be used – Second, when children in the target age range are not capable of completing a PRO measure, an informant-reported measure may be used – Informant-reported measures should assess observable content as much as possible
4. Ensure that the instrument is designed and formatted appropriately for the target age group	– Health-related vocabulary and reading level – Response scale – Recall period – Length of instrument – Pictorial representations – Formatting – Administration approaches – Electronic data collection (ePRO)
5. Consider cross-cultural issues	– Content validity and measurement approach of a paediatric PRO instrument will need to be reexamined within each new culture

7.5.3 Nonclinical assessments

The question about invasive or intrusive assessments can be tricky. To protect adolescents from invasive punctures for blood testing, some protocols required adolescent girls to perform repeated urine tests during a clinical trial. This, of course, is not invasive but can be perceived as very intrusive for some adolescents or their family. Recruitment could suffer as the informed consent and assent processes may trigger understandable concerns that could be alleviated by adding a serum pregnancy test to the standard biological safety assessments.

As a general rule, pain, fear, and distress must be prevented and minimised when unavoidable. If hospitalisation is required, depending on the nature and duration of the study, parents should be able to stay with their children overnight.

7.5.4 Timing of study procedures

Flexibility should be the rules. In some cases it can be acceptable to conduct study procedures during school hours, while for others, it will not be an option. Study procedures should impact as little as possible to children social lives, and assents have been denied by adolescents considering that they were interfering to an unacceptable extend to their sports activities, musical education, or school schedule.

7.5.5 Appropriate formulations

As evidenced by the WHO campaign, 'Make Medicines Child Size', paediatric formulations can create numerous challenges. This can lead to investigators not pursuing some research projects, and some initiatives have been developed to circumvent these issues. For instance, for investigator-led clinical trials within England, the National Institute of Health Research Clinical Research Network: Children (CRN: Children) provides support for formulations and pharmacy-related issues to researchers planning and setting up paediatric clinical trials (Wan et al., 2016).

For pharmaceutical companies, age-appropriate formulations are usually part of the regulatory commitments. However, commercial formulations do not have to be finalised for clinical trials; what is essential is to ensure that clinical studies will be conducted with specific age-appropriate formulations. Oral formulations are the preferred route for administration in paediatric patients, but some solid oral dosage forms that are used in adults may be inappropriate for children, and this can be an issue when an active reference, that is, for instance, considered as the current golden standard, does not have an optimal formulation available for use as clinical trial supplies.

7.5.6 Long-term care

Clinical studies cannot be performed without thinking of mid- to long-term management care, and when studies in child and adolescent psychiatry are conducted, this should be connected with the guarantee of the availability of appropriate healthcare for participants after they finish participating in the study.

Of course, long-term use of any drug in paediatric population raises specific concerns for safety and tolerability, and therefore long-term safety studies are usually needed. However, they should not be the only option for continuing providing drugs. Some ethics committees and some countries consider this as an ethical requirement.

7.5.7 Specialised settings

Paediatric trials need to involve specialists who know well the study population, who are empathic and sensitive to a child's needs and fears, and who have received study-specific training. Actually, it is usually easier to train investigating sites on study procedures than on study population.

Specific attention should be given to child-friendly environments.

7.5.8 Clear involvement of families, caregivers, and children

Everything should be done to ensure that clear information has been provided to children, adolescents, parents, and caregivers to ensure optimal patient and family involvement. Specific attention should be given to school attendance during trials and to parent's attendance (dependent on work and hour constraints). Avoiding hospitalisation is a must, and out-patient studies should be favoured.

Rescue therapy should be considered and discussed with parents, but rescue therapies should be precisely assessed as they can potentially bias randomized clinical trials and even turn to be unethical, as actually a child's involvement in a clinical trial could be more ethical than offering a therapeutic rescue without discontinuing the child's participation. Study design should be very precise in this respect (Holubkov et al., 2009).

Considering that global clinical trials are now the rule rather than the exception, cultural aspects should also be taken into consideration when designing paediatric programmes.

7.5.9 Slow recruitment

Recruitment is almost always slower compared with adult studies except in ADHD, not only due to demographic or epidemiological reasons but also owing to multifactorial factors relating to doctor, parent, child, and trial; one of the key factors is that the threshold for gaining consent is often higher and more complicated (and will be the focus of the next chapter). This needs to be taken into account when planning the study. As speed is always an issue, realistic expectations have to be understood before starting any trial, and feasibility should be discussed not only with investigating sites but also with patients' organisations or representatives.

7.5.10 Data monitoring committee/data safety monitoring board

Data monitoring committee (DMC) or data safety monitoring board (DSMB) should always be considered, even in noncritical indications. They are now part of good practice in paediatric clinical trials, especially as children are not capable of expressing themselves in the same way as adults do. Their role is discussed in the chapter focusing on safety.

Interestingly, there are innovative approaches to support decision-making process including modern statistical approaches including Bayesian approach.

7.6 Conclusion

This topic of study design and methodology is complex, potentially controversial but cannot be dissociated from science and ethics. We have presented in this first of three chapters some of the points we believe are crucial to consider when developing paediatric protocols. We advocate in this chapter to further involve patients and families. Of course, our perspective remains based on our personal experiences, does not pretend to be exhaustive, and can be criticised for these reasons, but we believe that this chapter illustrates probably the best what Rabelais was telling in 1532: Science without conscience is but the ruin of the soul.

The following two chapters will focus on the specificities of paediatric recruitment and the issue of indiscriminative efficacy trials and placebo effects in paediatric psychopharmacology.

References

Auby, P., 2018. Development of Medicines in Child and Adolescent Psychiatry: Industry Perspective. Regulatory Spotlight Session. Presentation on behalf of the Efpia at the ECNP Barcelona.

Bar-Shalom, D., Rose, K. (Eds.), 2014. Pediatric Formulations: A Roadmap. Springer.

Bridge, J.A., Birmaher, B., Iyengar, S., Barbe, R.P., Brent, D.A., 2009. Placebo response in randomized controlled trials of antidepressants for pediatric major depressive disorder. Am. J. Psychiatry 166, 42–49.

Caron, C., Rutter, M., 1991. Comorbidity in child psychopathology: concepts, issues and research strategies. J. Child Psychol. Psychiatry 32, 1063–1080.

Cooper, N.J., Jones, D.R., Sutton, A.J., 2005. The use of systematic reviews when designing studies. Clin. Trials 2 (3), 260–264.

Emslie, G.J., Ryan, N.D., Wagner, K.D., 2005. Major depressive disorder in children and adolescents: clinical trial design and antidepressant efficacy. J. Clin. Psychiatry 66 (Suppl. 7), 14–20.

Fava, M., Evins, A.E., Dorer, D.J., Schoenfeld, D.A., 2003. The problem of the placebo response in clinical trials for psychiatric disorders: culprits, possible remedies, and a novel study design approach. Psychother. Psychosom. 72 (3), 115–127. Review. Erratum in: Psychother. Psychosom. 2004 73(2), 123.

Goodyer, I.M., Dubicka, B., Wilkinson, P., Kelvin, R., Roberts, C., Byford, S., et al., 2007. Selective serotonin reuptake inhibitors (SSRIs) and routine specialist care with and without cognitive behaviour therapy in adolescents with major depression: randomized controlled trial. BMJ 335, 142. Epub 7 Jun 2007.

Goodyer, I.M., Reynolds, S., Barrett, B., Byford, S., Dubicka, B., Hill, J., Holland, F., Kelvin, R., Midgley, N., Roberts, C., Senior, R., Target, M., Widmer, B., Wilkinson, P., Fonagy, P., 2017. Cognitive–behavioural therapy and short-term psychoanalytic psychotherapy versus brief psychosocial intervention in adolescents with unipolar major depression (IMPACT): a multicentre, pragmatic, observer-blind, randomised controlled trial. Heath Technol Assess 21 (12), 1–94. https://doi.org/10.3310/hta21120.

Hazell, P., O'Connell, D., Heathcote, D., Robertson, J., Henry, D., 1995. Efficacy of tricyclic drugs in treating child and adolescent depression: a meta-analysis. BMJ 310, 897–901.

Holubkov, R., Dean, J.M., Berger, J., 2009. Is 'rescue' therapy ethical in randomized controlled trials? Pediatr. Crit. Care Med. 10 (4), 431–438.

Kaufman, J., Birmaher, B., Axelson, D., Perepletchikova, F., Brent, D., Kiddie, R.N., 2016. Sads-Present and Lifetime Version – DSM-5 (K-SADS-PL – DSM-5). https://www.kennedykrieger.org/sites/default/files/library/documents/faculty/ksads-dsm-5-screener.pdf.

Matza, L.S., Patrick, D.L., Riley, A.W., Alexander, J.J., Rajmil, L., Pleil, A.M., Bullinger, M., 2013. Pediatric patient-reported outcome instruments for research to support medical product labeling: report of the ISPOR PRO good research practices for the assessment of children and adolescents task force. Value Health 16 (4), 461–479.

Persico, A.M., Arango, C., Buitelaar, J.K., Correll, C.U., Glennon, J.C., Hoekstra, P.J., Moreno, C., Vitiello, B., Vorstman, J., Zuddas, A., the European Child and Adolescent Clinical Psychopharmacology Network, 2015. Unmet needs in paediatric psychopharmacology: present scenario and future perspectives. Eur. Neuropsychopharmacol. 25 (10), 1513–1531.

Poznanski, E.O., Mokros, H.B., 1996. Children's Depression Rating Scale – Revised (CDRS-R): Manual. Western Psychological Services, Los Angeles, CA.

Wan, M., Al Hashimi, A., Batchelor, H., 2016. Pharmacy and formulation support for paediatric clinical trials in England. Int. J. Pharma. 511 (2), 1163–1168.

Youngstrom, E.A., Findling, R.L., Youngstrom, J.K., Calabrese, J.R., 2005. Toward an evidence-based assessment of pediatric bipolar disorder. J. Clin. Child Adolesc. Psychol. 34 (3), 433–448.

Further reading

Auby, P., 2014. The European Union Pediatric legislation: impact on pharmaceutical research in pediatric populations. Clin. Invest. 4 (11), 1013–1019.

Doros, G., Pencina, M., Rybin, D., Meisner, A., Fava, M., 2003. A repeated measures model for analysis of continuous outcome in sequential parallel comparison design studies. Stat. Med. 32 (16), 2767–2789.

https://www.ich.org/home.html.

https://www.ich.org/products/guidelines.html.

https://www.transceleratebiopharmainc.com/assets/common-protocol-template/.

Special challenges in paediatric recruitment

Karel Allegaert [a,b], Philippe Auby [c]
[a]Department of Pediatrics, Division of Neonatology, Erasmus MC-Sophia Children's Hospital, Rotterdam, The Netherlands, [b]Department of Development and Regeneration, KU Leuven, Leuven, Belgium, [c]Otsuka Pharmaceutical Development & Commercialisation Europe, Frankfurt am Main, Germany

8.1 Introduction

By virtue of their developmental and cognitive abilities, children are considered to be a vulnerable population, depending on adults for protection. This is also true when considering their participation in a clinical trial. In addition to adaptations of the clinical protocol design (e.g. drug formulation, dosing, sampling strategy, and clinical indication), recruitment and retention strategies, incentives, and the process to obtain informed consent must be adapted appropriately for children.

8.2 Why an ethical sound paediatric recruitment strategy should be the rule?

The currently limited experience with paediatric recruitment is the current result of a historical pendulum movement. During the 18th and 19th centuries, children were often viewed as 'property' of their parents or legal representatives and frequently recruited for research, mainly in the field of infectious diseases and vaccines with subsequent protection since the mid-20th century, formalised in the Helsinki declaration. Unfortunately, protecting children (and pregnant women following the Softenon event) got translated to excluding these populations from clinical trials, resulting in the concept of 'therapeutic orphans'.

The danger of simple extrapolation of findings as collected in adults to the paediatric population has been well recognised, and some of the anecdotal errors (chloramphenicol in neonates, formulation errors, human immunodeficiency virus (HIV)-related drugs in children, and inappropriate questionnaires) are well known in the paediatric community. Differences due to differences in physiological responses to disease, in disease characteristics, in treatment modalities, or due to the ontogeny of drug disposition necessitate the collection of age-specific observations at various stages of paediatric maturation.

At present, either unlicensed or off-label administration of drugs is frequent and in part depends on disease severity. Ironically, unlicensed or off-label administration of drugs is most frequent (60%–80%) the most critically ill patients (neonatal and paediatric intensive care), still 40%–60% in a paediatric hospital setting and 20%–40 % in ambulatory care. This attitude is not without risk: unknown adverse events, poorly established efficacy, hazardous dose calculation, and inappropriate formulation. This problem also exists in the specific field of child and adolescent psychiatry and mental health as mentioned by Zito et al. (2008).

Both US and EU paediatric regulations can be a strong incentive to generate the data patients, clinicians, and the society need, that is, more data on the effective use of drugs in children (Auby, 2014). However, to ensure a successful impact of these regulations, numerous challenges have to be considered including the specific challenges related to recruitment in paediatric clinical studies.

A stakeholder approach might be an appropriated way to understand the current position of all the relevant contributors needed to turn the current EU regulation into an effective tool. Caregivers have to develop clinical research networks and will have to develop specific clinical research skills in addition to their clinical care. Knowledge of parental perceived barriers and incentives is of relevance to facilitate recruitment and retention, while the child neither is 'an innocent bystander' of a trial based on the concept of 'assent'. In paediatric research, the trial design probably affects recruitment to a greater extent compared with adult studies. In general, if a study is designed well, with a clear clinical question with which parents/children can identify, they are likely to consider participation.

Just like children are not small adults, paediatric studies are not just subgroup-adult studies. Effective, open communication with all stakeholders involved will most likely result in the initial idea behind this EU regulation, that is, ethically correct, practically feasible, scientifically sound, and economically reasonable studies are the most effective way to provide the children with the appropriated drugs and treatment they need.

Importantly, effective implementation of these regulations necessitates the collaboration of all stakeholders involved in the search for an adapted 'good clinical practice' approach: that is, ethically correct, practically feasible, scientifically sound, and economic reasonable. It is to be anticipated that open communication and confidence between the various stakeholders (the community including patients and their parents, academia, industry, and government) will be crucial to achieving the common goal, that is, to reduce off-label use of medicines in children so that their medical treatment is based on evidence and the understanding of developmental physiology. From an industrial or clinical research organisation point of view, this will necessitate networking and collaboration with healthcare professionals, initially and mainly trained for clinical care and parents/patients. For healthcare professionals, this will necessitates readiness to develop clinical research networks and specific clinical research skills in addition to the clinical caretaking of patients. A stakeholder approach might be an excellent way to understand the current position of all the relevant contributors needed to turn paediatric regulations into effective tools.

8.3 Stakeholders involved in paediatric recruitment and retention

8.3.1 Healthcare professionals

Several techniques have been used to recruit for participation in paediatric trials. Advertisements, mailings, or posters have not been found to be successful. The digital revolution may be useful to provide better communication channels.

However, in any case, partnerships with health professionals in various paediatric settings are perceived to be the most effective way to facilitate recruitment and subsequent retention (Caldwell et al., 2004). This is, in general, a somewhat different approach compared with phase I studies but relatively similar to phase II/III studies in adults. For instance, in Europe, taking the paediatric regulatory framework into account with its specific emphasis on drug research in sick children, linkage with learned societies, research organisations, and academia is needed, and partnerships have to be further developed. The recent initiative in the United States by the Institute for Advanced Clinical Trials for Children (iACT for Children) and a similar European initiative (Care 4 Children, C4C) hereby reflect the willingness to build research capacity for paediatric research and develop clinical trial infrastructure.

Most parents have a trusting relationship with 'their' healthcare provider (e.g. paediatrician and paediatric nurse) and are more willing to follow the healthcare provider's recommendation. Besides the general concept of 'confidence' in the healthcare provider, successful recruitment into paediatric trials is also enhanced if parents perceive a threat to the personal health of their child for which the study might be helpful such as the development of a new medication related to the child's diagnosis (Caldwell et al., 2004; Tait et al., 2004, Knox and Burkhart, 2007). This has been illustrated by a French study in cohorts of children with cancer or HIV infection. The possibility to receive the most advanced treatments together with the confidence in the medical team was their highest motivations for participation (Tait et al., 2004; Knox and Burkhart, 2007).

External sponsors have to be aware that barriers at the level of healthcare professionals also exist, although there have been fewer studies on this issue. Paediatricians acknowledge that unawareness, time and financial constraints, difficulties with the formal requirements, and concerns on the doctor–patient relationship may be barriers (Caldwell et al., 2002). Better education of the medical community is needed about the rationale and benefits of trials and the potential dangers of using healthcare interventions that have not been appropriately studied. A win–win setting by providing training on Good Clinical Practice (GCP) guidelines should be considered since one had to be aware that the clinical care–patient relationship is different from the clinical scientist–patient relationship. Ensure that all co-workers of a given study are aware of the methodology of GCP before the start of the study. Once healthcare providers are aware of the relevance of recruitment and retention, (s)he may also serve as a filter to preconsider potential patients for recruitment. The recruitment through healthcare professionals appears the most effective approach, but this is a relatively vulnerable concept of which both parents and healthcare professionals are not always aware of. In the complex relationship between parents and physician(s), there is a risk of unrealised obligations and emotional subordination. Moreover, this may not be perceived by either party (Tait et al., 2004; Knox and Burkhart, 2007).

8.3.2 Parents

In paediatric trials, parental consent is required and an absolute prerequisite (Caldwell et al., 2004; Van Stuijvenberg et al., 1998). Knowledge of parental perceived barriers and incentives is therefore of relevance to facilitate paediatric recruitment and retention. In its essence, 'if a trial is designed well with a clear clinical question with which parents can identify, then they are likely to consider participation' (Van Stuijvenberg et al., 1998; Tait et al., 2003, 2005).

In a study on the motivations of British parents to consent for participation of their child in a study on the effectiveness of oral versus intravenous antibiotics for community-acquired pneumonia, questionnaires were mailed to assess what motivates parents to consent, their feelings on consent and participation, and the factors that would influence their decision to take part in a future study. The most important reason given by parents was the anticipated benefit to all children in the future and contribution to clinical knowledge (57%) or perceived benefit for their own child (18%). Thirteen percent participated because the doctor asked for and 7% because there was no reason not to participate (Sammons et al., 2007). Similar results were reported by a Dutch group which analysed the reasons for participation in a trial on the administration of ibuprofen for secondary prevention of febrile convulsions (Van Stuijvenberg et al., 1998).

Information on motivations to participate in research may enable researchers and sponsors to tailor the process of recruitment and consent to the needs and perceptions of parents and their children. In a recent systematic review to assess motivating and discouraging factors for parents and their children, most mentioned motivating factors for parents are perceived health benefit, altruism, trust in research, and relation to the researcher. For children, these factors were health benefit, altruism, and increasing comfort. In contrast, perceived risks, distrust in research, practical aspects, and interference with the routine daily life were most frequently mentioned as discouraging factors by the parents. Burden and disruption of daily life, feeling like a 'guinea pig', and fear of risks were most commonly mentioned by children as discouraging factors (Tromp et al., 2016).

The sense of urgency is less often perceived as an issue in paediatric psychopharmacology, but the feelings of unanticipated medical conditions are often verbalised by parents; the specific setting of neonatal research where indeed there is almost always such sense of urgency and/or unanticipated medical condition can give additional insights. In this specific population, parents want to be involved in the decision to enter a research project; even those who felt significant added stress by the research project agree to consent for societal benefit, personal gain, and the perception of no harm. Refuse of consent is mainly because of the risk of harm, antiexperimentation beliefs, or clinician approach. Parents would agree to their child being in more than one trial and do find some of the concepts of trials difficult to understand but mainly rely on verbal explanation and information sheets in making decisions (McKechnie and Gill, 2006).

Understanding the informed consent document by the parents is crucial. Some of the predictors of understanding are parent based (level of education), but some of these factors can be improved. Readability and processability are therefore crucial (Tait et al., 2003, 2005). Most informed consent documents are typically written well above the recommended eighth-grade reading level. Besides the readability, the processability of the information (e.g. layout, mental images, and context clues) can further improve the informed consent procedure and subsequent compliance. The additional verbal disclosure further improves this procedure. Parents felt essential that they were able to discuss the study protocol and their concerns with research nurses before consent was provided (Tait et al., 2003, 2005).

8.3.3 Child

The child is not an innocent bystander in paediatric trials as reflected in the concept of 'assent'. The notion of 'assent' is recognised in the declaration of Helsinki ('when a subject deemed legally incompetent, such as a minor child, is able to give assent to decision about participation in research, the investigator must obtain that assent in addition to the consent of the legally authorised representative') and in European guidelines (EMEA, 2012). The evaluation of whether or not a child can give assent should not only be based on chronological age but also depend on other factors as the developmental stage or intellectual capacities. Separate information sheets for adults and children should be used to provide age-appropriate information (Tait et al., 2007).

In a semistructured interview with children attending outpatient paediatric clinics, most children recognised that there were risks involved with participating in clinical trials, but views on payment were more different (Cherrill et al., 2007). In Europe, it is not acceptable to pay children for participating in research, and similarly, it is considered inappropriate to recruit healthy children for pharmacokinetic studies.

Acute illness is more favourable for recruitment, while the extent of disruption of the 'regular' routine is one of the most critical issues to consider. Issues of convenience (increased clinic visits and transportation difficulties) and concerns about the demands of the intensive treatment (e.g. increased injections) were the predominant reasons for trial refusal in a cohort of adolescents with diabetes mellitus (Caldwell et al., 2004; Knox and Burkhart, 2007). Following initial recruitment, retention is another issue to be considered. Flexible scheduling with limited disruption of the child's daily routine including education, extracurricular activities, and time with their peers seems crucial. Home visits to accommodate for these circumstances should be considered and mainly depend on the type of study. As mentioned in the 'Patient's voice' chapter, the International Children's Advisory Network (iCAN) may hereby serve as a nice illustration of capacity and expertise building of children to improve paediatric healthcare by providing children and the families a voice in health care, including clinical research and innovations in medicine. This network contains several chapters across the globe and became a relevant stakeholder. A limited number of people with whom a single participant has contacts further improve retention.

8.4   Trial design

In paediatric research, the trial design probably affects recruitment to a greater extent than in adult studies. In general, the more complex and the more invasive, the harder to recruit. To enhance recruitment, any study should aim to involve patients as close to the clinical situation as possible. As mentioned earlier, 'if a trial is designed well with a clear clinical question with which parents can identify, then they are likely to consider participation'. Potential risks and inconveniences perceived to be of additional relevance in children include discomfort, inconvenience, pain, fear, separation from parents and family, effects on growing and developing organs, and size or volume of biological samples (EMEA, 2006). Early mentioned structures like the iCAN initiative may hereby provide relevant guidance.

Pragmatic trial design, which does not impose a burden of treatment; testing; and monitoring beyond routine clinical care are designed to obviate additional risks for trial participation. Use of placebo in children is more restricted than in adults because children cannot consent (Caldwell et al., 2004; Knox and Burkhart, 2007; EMEA, 2012). Placebo should not be used when it means withholding effective treatment. As the level of evidence in favour of an effective treatment increases, the ethical justification for placebo decreased. Placebo use is not equivalent to the absence of treatment but could be used on top of standard care. As many medicines used in children have not been adequately assessed and authorised, medicinal products without marketing authorisation may be considered suitable as controls if they represent the evidence-based standard of care. For parents, a placebo-controlled trial approach is assessed to have a higher risk/benefit.

8.5   Discussion: paediatric trials on trial

Just like children are not small adults, paediatric studies are not just subgroup-adult studies. Investigators should employ innovative approaches to facilitate recruitment and retention of children in clinical research. Effective strategies likely mainly depend on partnerships between research initiators/sponsors, the paediatric healthcare providers, patients, and their parents (Ramet, 2005).

Key planning details include input from caregivers on patient volumes, including nursing staff, and one should ensure that all caregivers are aware that the clinical care/patient relationship is entirely similar to the clinical research/patient relationship. Parents of sick children are aware that well-designed clinical studies are needed. This awareness should be further enforced. A readable and understandable consent form is crucial in the communication with parents since it is essential: if there is a well-designed study, with a clear clinical question, parents will consider participation

(Van Stuijvenberg et al., 1998). Children should be informed on the recruitment in an age-appropriate approach, and the concept of 'assent' is crucial. Children are aware of potential risks and can make balanced decisions (Cherrill et al., 2007). Potential risks and inconveniences perceived to be of additional relevance in children include discomfort, inconvenience, pain, fear, separation from parents and family, effects on growing and developing organs, and size or volume of biological samples. Pragmatic trial design is therefore crucial. Not to impose a burden of treatment, testing and monitoring beyond routine clinical care obviate additional risks for trial participation (Caldwell et al., 2004; Knox and Burkhart, 2007; EMEA, 2012; Cherrill et al., 2007). Communication is, therefore, crucial and should be started at the moment of trial design, not at the moment of initiation of the clinical part of the trial.

Effective communication between regulators, pharmaceutical companies, clinicians, and other key stakeholders is needed. The dialogue between these partners in health care needs to be strengthened, and the available learned societies and dedicated research networks should take their responsibilities. Following the Paediatric Regulation request, the European Medicines Agency (EMA) has built and further developed a European network of existing national and European networks, investigators, and groups with specific expertise in the performance of studies in the paediatric population (Enpr-EMA, n.d.). The first step was to identify all existing networks, groups, and investigators with specific paediatric expertise to facilitate this communication process. Finally, we have to be aware that drug development priorities tend to be driven primarily by economic influences, but academia or the public should consider in a balanced approach the primary needs of drug research for children in the world.

8.6 Conclusion

The concept of paediatric trials itself is on trial. Effective, open communication with all stakeholders involved will most likely result in the initial idea behind this concept, that is, ethically correct, practically feasible, scientifically sound, and economic reasonable studies are the most effective way to provide the children with the appropriated drugs and treatment they need.

References

Auby, P., 2014. The European Union Pediatric legislation: impact on pharmaceutical research in pediatric populations. Clin. Invest. 4 (11), 1013–1019.

Caldwell, P.H., Butow, P.N., Craig, J.C., 2002. Paediatricians' attitudes toward randomized controlled trials involving children. J. Pediatr. 141, 798–803.

Caldwell, P.H., Murphy, S.B., Butow, P.N., Craig, J.C., 2004. Clinical trials in children. Lancet 364, 803–811.

Cherrill, J., Hudson, H., Cocking, C., Unsworth, V., Franck, L., McIntyre, J., Choonara, I., 2007. Clinical trials: the viewpoint of children. Arch. Dis. Child. 92, 712–713.

EMEA, 2006. http://www.ema.europa.eu/docs/en_GB/document_library/Scientific_guideline/2009/09/.
EMEA, 2012. http://www.ema.europa.eu/docs/en_GB/document_library/Report/2012/10/WC500134407.pdf.
Enpr-EMA, http://www.ema.europa.eu/ema/index.jsp?curl=pages/partners_and_networks/general/general_content_000303.jsp&mid=WC0b01ac05801df74a.
Knox, C.A., Burkhart, P.V., 2007. Issues related to children participating in clinical research. J. Pediatr. Nurs. 22, 310–318.
McKechnie, L., Gill, A.B., 2006. Consent for neonatal research. Arch. Dis. Child. Fetal Neonatal Ed. 91, F374–F376.
Ramet, J., 2005. What the paediatricians need – the launch of paediatric research in Europe. Eur. J. Pediatr. 164, 263–265.
Sammons, H.M., Atkinson, M., Choonara, I., Stephenson, T., 2007. What motivates British parents to consent for research? A questionnaire study. BMC Pediatr. 7, 12.
Tait, A.R., Voepel-Lewis, T., Malviya, S., 2003. Do they understand? Parental consent for children participating in clinical anesthesia and surgery research. Anesthesiology 98, 603–608.
Tait, A.R., Voepel-Lewis, T., Malviya, S., 2004. Factors that influence parents' assessments of risks and benefits of research involving their children. Pediatrics 113, 727–732.
Tait, A.R., Voepel-Lewis, T., Malviya, S., Philipson, S.J., 2005. Improving the readability and processability of a paediatric informed consent: effects on parents' understanding. Arch. Pediatr. Adolesc. Med. 159, 347–352.
Tait, A.R., Voepel-Lewis, T., Malviya, S., 2007. Presenting research information to children: a tale of two methods. Anesth. Analg. 105, 358–364.
Tromp, K., Zwaan, C.M., van de Vathorst, S., 2016. Motivations of children and their parents to participate in drug research: a systematic review. Eur. J. Pediatr. 175 (5), 599–612.
Van Stuijvenberg, M., Suur, M.H., de Vos, S., Tjiang, G.C., Steyerberg, E.W., Derksen-Lubsen, G., Moll, H.A., 1998. Informed consent, parental awareness, and reasons for participating in a randomised controlled study. Arch. Dis. Child. 79, 120–125.
Zito, J.M., Derivan, A.T., Kratochvil, C.J., Safer, D.J., Fegert, J.M., Greenhill, L.L., 2008. Off-label psychopharmacologic prescribing for children: history supports close clinical monitoring. Child Adolesc. Psychiatry Ment. Health 2, 24.

Further reading

http://conect4children.org/news/press-release-launch-of-the-c4c-project/.
https://www.iactc.org/.

In Memoriam: Professor Dr. Klaudius Siegfried

Professor Doctor Klaudius Siegfried's final academic contribution was to this book. I was invited to write something in honor of his memory, and I am very proud to have done so, as it provided me with an opportunity to reminisce about my old friend and colleague.

Prof. Dr. Siegfried studied psychology, physiology, and psychiatry/neurology at Goethe University Frankfurt (Main) and completed his clinical training at Frankfurt Medical School. His doctoral thesis was on psychological diagnostics. He later completed a second, 'Habilitation', thesis on clinical profiles of antidepressants with different pharmacological properties, as part of his qualification as a university professor in Germany. In parallel with his distinguished CNS career in the pharmaceutical industry, he rose through the academic ranks from lecturer to full professor and spent over 35 years teaching at Goethe University Frankfurt (Main) and, more recently, at the University of Ulm (Germany). He taught classes on mental disorders, clinical neuropsychology, clinical psychopharmacology, clinical trial methodologies, and rating scale assessments. He also supervised doctoral theses. While German was his mother tongue, he also spoke English fluently and was conversant in French, Italian, and Spanish and knew some Latin and ancient Greek. He traveled extensively in the United States and enjoyed spending holidays there with his family.

His distinguished pharmaceutical industry career included therapeutic, scientific, strategic, and operational aspects of international drug development across all major CNS indications. He interacted regularly with academic and key opinion leaders in CNS research and development, presented to and negotiated with global regulatory authorities (EMEA, FDA, etc.), and oversaw planning and operations for CNS studies in the Americas, Europe, Asia, South Africa, and Australia. Following his clinical training, Prof. Dr. Siegfried's first industry position was in the Medical and Clinical Development Department of Hoechst Pharmaceuticals in Frankfurt (Main), Germany. He began as a global clinical project manager (1985–2000) with therapeutic, scientific, drug development, strategic, and operational responsibilities. In September of 2000, Prof. Dr. Siegfried joined ICON Clinical Research as a director and, only 1 year later, was promoted to Sr. Director. By 2006, he was the vice president for CNS Research and Global Leader of the CNS Therapeutic Area. His responsibilities had now shifted to include all of ICON's global CNS programs, providing oversight of protocol writing, protocol review, rating scale training, and study feasibility evaluations. His scientific advice was sought after by many sponsors across global CNS Drug Development Programs.

As he neared retirement age, Prof. Dr. Siegfried expressed some concern over how he would handle the transition from always being on the go and constantly being sought after, to the lack of many responsibilities that goes along with retirement. Would he feel useless and forgotten? His retirement would only be part time, as he continued to consult with ICON on scientific issues and provided therapeutic training and support. In retirement, he also continued to give lectures and to lead seminars at the University of Frankfurt (Main) and at Ulm University. He maintained his professional involvement in several important scientific organisations that included the German Association for Neuropsychopharmacology and Pharmacopsychiatry (AGNP), British Association for Psychopharmacology (BAP), European College of Neuropsychopharmacology (ECNP), Collegium Internationale Neuropsychopharmacologicum (CINP), and Collegium Internationale Psychiatriae Scalarum (CIPS). He also continued his academic writing and was excited about being asked to contribute to this book. Prof. Dr. Siegfried derived much pleasure from scientific writing and discussions. He wrote over 60 scientific publications and, for over 13 years, served on editorial boards as an advisory editor for several scientific journals and books.

In addition to having been a highly respected scholar, Prof. Dr. Siegfried was a generous man. He would freely give of his valuable time to anyone who asked for his help and truly enjoyed teaching others. If you were lucky enough to spend an evening with him in a pub, the conversation would likely turn to philosophy, psychology, existentialism, and good wine. He loved exchanging ideas with friends over a glass of wine. He will be missed by his family, his colleagues, and his friends from all over the world. Goodbye Klaudius, and thank you for your many scientific contributions and for being a dear friend.

Paul Michael Ramirez
Long Island University, Brooklyn, NY, United States

The issue of indiscriminative efficacy trials and placebo effects in paediatric psychopharmacology

Klaudius Siegfried[†]
Goethe Univ. Frankfurt, Frankfurt, Germany

9.1 Introduction

Over the last approximately 20 years, paediatric experts and regulatory agencies have repeatedly emphasised the need of more clinical studies in children and adolescents that meet the highest scientific standards and provide data required for evidence-based drug treatment recommendations (Persico et al., 2015). Many drugs approved for adults are used in children based on off-label prescriptions, without sufficient paediatric data. Therefore regulatory authorities (the US Food and Drug Administration, FDA; the European Medicines Agency, EMA) have been trying to encourage and enforce the conduct of such studies by providing incentives for pharmaceutical industry (e.g. extended market exclusivity for drugs) and requiring paediatric studies for drugs newly approved for adults (e.g. in the United States: the 'Paediatric Rule' and 'Paediatric Study Incentive', 'Best Pharmaceuticals for Children Act', and 'Paediatric Research Equity Act'; the 'Paediatric Regulation' by the Council of the European Union) (Persico et al., 2015; Yao, 2013).

This chapter will focus on an important group of hurdles and impediments that are blocking the attainment of the goal of evidence-based treatment recommendations in paediatric psychopharmacology, the issue of indiscriminative efficacy studies which falsely suggest no differences between active drug and placebo. Strong placebo effects are not the only but a major reason for such studies. This issue slows down and impedes the development of new, especially innovative drugs, has a negative impact on therapeutic progress, and deprives clinicians of possibly valuable treatment options. The objectives of this article will be

(a) to review available evidence that describes and illustrates the issue caused by false-negative efficacy studies and placebo effects in clinical psychopharmacology,
(b) to compare the magnitude and scope of this issue in adult and paediatric studies and point out its particular relevance for paediatric psychopharmacology,
(c) to provide an overview of the known and hypothesised sources of false-negative indiscriminative studies with special focus on factors of placebo effects, and
(d) to discuss and recommend measures likely to help reducing the number of false-negative indiscriminative studies and the magnitude of placebo effects.

[†]Deceased.

9.2 Basic concepts, definitions, and methodological considerations

The core issues discussed in this chapter are difficulties in demonstrating statistically significant differences between placebo and active drug treatment. Statistical significance is a necessary (but not sufficient) prerequisite of clinical relevance. The basis of all of the following presentations, discussions, and recommendations are therefore *placebo-controlled studies*. The requirement of placebo-controlled clinical studies in psychiatric indications has never been uncontroversial, especially for paediatric populations. Specifically, besides possible ethical concerns, doubts have been raised if these types of studies do not perhaps artificially create a problem that would otherwise not exist. However, the majority of clinical experts, methodologists, and regulatory authorities consider a comparison of a new experimental drug against placebo as a necessary, indispensable requirement for the valid unequivocal demonstration of efficacy in all therapeutic areas where the expected treatment effects are likely to be only small to moderate in magnitude and placebo effects substantial and variable, varying across different settings and studies (Leber, 1991; Montgomery, 1999). Unfortunately, these qualifications apply to most, if not all, areas of psychopharmacology and in particular to drug treatment in paediatric populations, as will be demonstrated in subsequent sections of this article. Studies that do not explicitly control for placebo effects ignore an important confounding factor in efficacy observations which makes it impossible to unambiguously allocate an observed clinical effect to the administered test drug. In extreme cases, this may lead to the approval and use of drugs with doubtful or clinically insignificant effects, which would be much more questionable from an ethical point of view than the conduct of (highly regulated and supervised) placebo-controlled studies. Open-labelled, noncomparative studies and randomised active-comparator studies do have their merits in the clinical investigation of new drugs, but their findings cannot be adequately interpreted without the results of some key ('pivotal') double-blind, randomised, placebo-controlled studies. Given the variability of placebo effects, non-significant differences or an 'equivalence' of test drugs and active comparators (or 'noninferiority' of the test drugs vs an active standard) leave the decisive efficacy question unanswered, namely, whether an 'equivalence' finding means that both drugs were equally efficacious or equally inefficacious.

In the introductory section, it was pointed out that the focus of this chapter will be *indiscriminative efficacy studies which falsely suggest no differences between an active drug and placebo*. This means that not all types of indiscriminative studies will be dealt with in the following but only a subgroup. There are indeed two broad classes of indiscriminative studies:

- Type 1 – Studies that cannot show superiority of (active) drug effects over placebo because the test drug is simply clinically inefficacious or has only minor, clinically irrelevant effects. These are called *'negative studies'*.
- Type 2 – Studies which fail to demonstrate a truly existing drug effect due to methodological or study conduct problems. These are called *'false-negative studies'*. They represent a subtype of *'failed studies'*.

In this chapter, we are only dealing with failed studies of the false-negative type. These studies have a lack of *'assay sensitivity'* (Leber, 1991), that is, are not sufficiently sensitive to differentiate between active drug and placebo effects. They are called 'failed' because they cannot adequately address the primary study question ('Is the drug tested superior to placebo?'). Their biggest practical problem is that post hoc explanations of their results (by methodological flaws, study conduct issues, etc.) can frequently only be based on plausible assumptions but not on convincing evidence. This is why these studies are also called *'nonconclusive'*. A convincing case can only be made when the study had a third treatment arm, a recognised (active) standard treatment, which could also not be separated from placebo, or when there are already other similar efficacy studies with the same test drug that were able to demonstrate efficacy. Unless there is such evidence, clinical researchers, sponsors, and regulators are facing a major dilemma in that they have difficulties making (informed) decisions on the value of a further development of the investigative drug.

False-negative indiscriminative studies are often caused by *placebo effects*. These occur in all clinical studies with psychotropic agents. The *'placebo (effect) issue'* is an issue of the *size (or magnitude)* of placebo effects and the *proportion of placebo responders* relative to active drug responders. The larger these effects and proportions, the higher the risk of false-negative indiscriminative studies. Increased placebo effects and elevated placebo responder rates frequently account for failed efficacy studies in psychopharmacology. They represent a major risk factor for false-negative indiscriminative studies. But they are not the only and also not a necessary reason. In some studies, efficacy can be demonstrated in spite of elevated placebo response rates, if the number of active drug responders is similarly elevated. So, it is not merely the pure size of the placebo effect and proportion of placebo responders that counts but the difference between the placebo and active drug group. In addition, the same difference between the active drug and treatment group can in one study be statistically significant but not in another. This is because indiscriminative false-negative studies can be caused by two major groups of factors (or both of them):

- The *magnitude of the difference between active drug and placebo group* (i.e. mean difference on a defined efficacy variable – or difference in the proportion of responders). This is driven, among other factors, by the size/magnitude of an improvement in the placebo group.
- The *size/magnitude of the variance of the outcome variable* (i.e. the size of the interindividual variability of the baseline–endpoint differences on a specified efficacy scale) within the treatment groups ('intragroup variances'). The larger the within-group ('intragroup') variances, in comparison with the between-group ('intergroup') variances, the greater the risk of an indiscriminative study outcome.

(Additional factors that determine the decision on statistical significance of a found effect are the size of type 1 and 2 errors, statistical power, and patient sample size.)

Finally, some clarifications and definitions appear to be necessary for an adequate understanding of the further discussion of placebo effects, their subtypes, and sources.

A *placebo* is a pharmacologically inert drug. An atheoretical definition of a *'placebo effect'* would simply describe it as an observed improvement in clinical condition of patients in the placebo arm of a clinical study. This definition has the merits of not including unproven, debatable hypothetical assumptions and facilitates an objective assessment (based on an operational definition). Its disadvantage is that it ignores the possibility of those improvements in clinical condition under active drug treatment that are not or at least not completely related to the pharmacological activity of the administered drug. Some researchers therefore prefer to define placebo effects in broader, less specific terms, namely, as an improvement in clinical condition due to *'unspecific'* (or *'nonspecific'*) factors (Finniss et al., 2010; Parellada et al., 2012). The weakness of this definition is not only its lacking operational rooting but also the fact that placebo effects are indeed not unspecific (Benedetti, 2014; Kirsch, 1997). They are driven by (a bundle of) specific factors. In ('pragmatic') clinical efficacy studies, these factors are usually *'unspecified'* (i.e. unplanned, uncontrolled, and therefore unidentifiable), which appears to be the background of the mentioned definition. Sometimes the concepts of *'placebo effect'* and *'placebo response'* are used interchangeably as synonyms. In this chapter, 'placebo *effect*' will refer to any observed improvement under placebo, whereas 'placebo *response*' is conceived as a *clinically significant* placebo effect. In clinical psychopharmacology studies, the latter is usually operationally defined as a 50% or greater improvement from baseline on a selected symptom scale. Alternatively, it is sometimes defined as ratings of 'much improved' or 'very much improved', compared with baseline, on the Clinical Global Impression of Improvement Scale (CGI-I: Guy, 1976).

An *observed* improvement under placebo can have different reasons. A first important step towards a differentiated understanding of placebo effects was the introduction of the distinction between *'true'* versus *'perceived'* placebo effects by Ernst and Resch (1995). In both cases, clinical observations and/or patient reports indicate improvements in clinical condition. However, whereas *'true effects'* refer to observations that reflect real changes in clinical conditions and are associated with alterations in neurobiological correlates, *'perceived effects'* are assessment artefacts that are merely suggesting an effect but not associated with real changes. Placebo effect researchers are inclined to argue that the earlier broad descriptive, operational concept of placebo effects (i.e. any improvement under placebo), which is mostly used by investigators of therapeutic drug studies, is inadequate because it includes a fairly large bundle of heterogeneous factor groups and is therefore not helpful in elucidating the mechanism(s) of these effects. These researchers prefer to restrict the definition of placebo effects to 'true' improvements due to *psychological* (and associated neurobiological) *processes in the psychosocial context of therapeutic settings* (Benedetti, 2014; Benedetti et al., 2005). Only these types of effects reflect patients' perception and evaluation of treatment and are the response of the brain to the therapeutic setting (Alphs et al., 2012). In our view, both the broader descriptive and the narrow and more specific concept have their justifications and merits, depending on the specific research interest and objective of a study. If the primary study objective is to analyze and distinguish the contribution of various factors of improvements in clinical condition under placebo, a narrow definition would certainly be more appropriate. For the usual pragmatic clinical efficacy studies, it will be, however, nearly impossible to identify specific factors of improvement under placebo and to distinguish 'true' from 'perceived' placebo effects. Study designs and procedures that allow an identification and control of different types of factors of improvement under placebo are likely to make clinical efficacy studies, which are anyway already fairly difficult to conduct, even more operationally complicated and endanger their feasibility. Obviously, it would be desirable to have, in addition, more studies that allow a precise identification of different sources of placebo effects. The majority of available data on placebo effects in psychopharmacology come from (pragmatic) efficacy studies and are based on retrospective (meta-)analyses and reviews. The latter have to accept a series of uncontrollable confounding factors which can make comparisons across studies and patient samples difficult. This is why their conclusions often need to remain hypothetical, and large data sets of comparable studies are required to give them an acceptable level of confidence. This qualifier naturally applies also to many data and conclusions presented in the following.

9.3 An illustration of the issue of placebo effects and false-negative indiscriminative efficacy results in paediatric psychopharmacology – Efficacy studies with antidepressants in depressive disorder

In this section the scope of the issue of false-negative indiscriminant studies and placebo effects will be illustrated by presenting an overview of the history and current status of clinical efficacy studies in the clinical investigation of antidepressants in major depressive disorder (MDD). An initial brief summary of findings in *adult studies* will serve as a background and reference for a better understanding of the specific impact of the issue in *paediatric psychopharmacology* which will be reviewed subsequently. MDD studies represent the area with the largest wealth of data on placebo response in clinical psychopharmacology, which makes them particularly suitable for such an illustration. For a correct understanding of this overview, it is essential to keep in mind that all studies mentioned here involved antidepressants with a finally established efficacy and regulatory approval for adult MDD.

In a review of 75 placebo-controlled clinical trials with antidepressants in *adult* MDD, published between 1981 and December 2000, the following mean responder rates were obtained (Walsh et al., 2002):

- *placebo* responder rate in adults: 29.7% (range: 12.5%–51.8%)
- *active drug* responder rate in adults: 50.1% (range: 31.8%–70.4%)

A comparison of the ranges of placebo and active drug response figures indicates a considerable overlap which is suggestive of a major risk of failed indiscriminative studies. This is confirmed by two additional publications issued in the same year. A survey of results from 45 clinical trials, submitted to the US Food and Drug Administration (FDA) between 1985 and 1997 and finally approved as efficacious in MDD, revealed that 52% of the trials failed to demonstrate (statistical) superiority of the investigational drug over placebo (Khan et al., 2002). A similar survey (Laughren, 2001) of 50 studies for eight finally approved antidepressants, submitted between 1987 and 1999 to the FDA, showed almost the same proportion of study failures

(46% or 23 from 50 trials). A recently published analysis of the FDA database for New Drug Application (NDA) registrations for antidepressants in adults (Khan et al., 2017) provided responder rates for trials with antidepressants submitted after the year 2000 that looked even more alarming than the earlier:

- *placebo* responder rate in adults: 36.2% (+6.6)
- *active* responder rate in adults: 46.6% (+7.0)

The question of temporal trends in responder rates will be discussed further in the succeeding text.

Although the number of studies conducted with *antidepressants in children and adolescents with MDD* is considerably smaller than those in adults, it is sufficiently large to allow comparisons between adult and paediatric populations. The following overview of placebo-controlled trials with antidepressants in paediatric MDD is based on two major sources, the first publication covering studies published between 1966 and 1992 and the second studies published between 1988 and 2006. These overviews will be supplemented by information on more recently conducted studies that were published after 2006.

1. *Survey of paediatric antidepressant studies (with tricyclic agents) published between 1966 and 1992* (Hazell et al., 1995)

    In a literature search conducted on randomised, double-blind, placebo-controlled studies in children and adolescents with MDD, using CDROM databases SilverPlatter Medline (1966–92) and Excerpta Medica (June 1974–92), the authors found 12 studies in which the following tricyclic antidepressants were tested: imipramine, amitriptyline, clomipramine, nortriptyline, and desipramine. This is a fairly representative set of tricyclics because it includes drugs with different antidepressant profile, with sedating and activating effects and with variations in mood or drive-enhancing properties. Two-thirds of the studies were conducted in children (with from 6 or 7 to 12 years of age) and one-third in adolescents. All but one trial indicated larger effects for active drug than placebo, but only in one study, which was conducted in *adolescents*, the difference between active drug and placebo was statistically significant. Response data were only provided in a subset of five studies. On average the response rate under placebo was 37% and under tricyclic antidepressants 38%. A metaanalysis of the 12 studies suggested an average effect size of 0.35 for the active drugs. According to Cohen (2008), this would indicate a small effect. However, Cohen's effect size needs to be interpreted with caution. Since it does not separate true variance from error variance (due to the unreliability of measures), especially effects classified as 'small effect sizes' do not necessarily indicate statistically significant changes.

2. *Survey of paediatric antidepressant studies with second-generation antidepressants published between January 1988 and July 2006* (Bridge et al., 2009)

    In a PubMed search, selecting randomised, placebo-controlled trials with *second-generation antidepressants in children and adolescents* (6–18 years of age) *with MDD*, that were published between January 1988 and July 2006, the authors found 12 clinical trials. In these the following eight antidepressants were tested (in parentheses: number of trials): fluoxetine (3), paroxetine (3), sertraline (3), citalopram (1), escitalopram (1), venlafaxine (1), nefazodone (1), and mirtazapine (1). Subjects' median age was 12.3 years (range: 12–15.6 years), and the median proportion of females was 0.53 (range: 0.46–0.68). The patient sample sizes per treatment arm ranged from 48 to 184 with a median size of 110. All studies used the Childrens' Depression Rating Scale (CDRS) (Poznanski et al., 1979) and

the Clinical Global Impression of Improvement (CGI-I) (Guy, 1976) as outcome measures. Response was defined by CGI-I classifications of either 'much improved' or 'very much improved'. Treatment duration was usually 8 weeks. The mean proportion of responders (based on CGI-I criteria) is listed in the succeeding text:
- *placebo* responder rate (all patients): 46% (range: 33%–57%)
  o in children (6–12 years): 49.6%
  o in adolescents (13–18 years): 44.5%
- *active drug* responder rate (all patients): 59% (range: 47%–69%)
  o in children: 58.4%
  o in adolescents: 61.5%

The difference in response rates for children and adolescents did not reach the level of statistical significance (using 95% confidence intervals). In a comment in the editorial of the journal, in which Bridge et al. (2009) analysis was published, Emslie (2009) emphasises that the variability of placebo response rates was the most important differentiator between positive and negative (or 'failed') studies. Further analyses by Bridge et al. (2009) indicated that the best predictor of placebo response rates was the number of study sites per trial. When one of the fluoxetine trials (Emslie et al., 1997), which showed a low rate of placebo response and had the lowest number of subjects per treatment arm ($n=48$ subjects), was excluded from the analysis, the age trend in placebo response between children and adolescents became significant.

The majority of paediatric MDD studies reviewed earlier was unable to demonstrate a significant superiority of active drug effects over placebo. Indeed, so far, fluoxetine is the only antidepressant which received a market approval by the FDA and EMA for both children and adolescents with MDD. The other exception is escitalopram. But, unlike fluoxetine, the latter has not been approved for children but for adolescents only. For all other antidepressants, indiscriminative efficacy results were obtained. Considering that all of these antidepressants have an established efficacy in adult MDD, most or a major subgroup of these indiscriminative studies are likely to be failed, false-negative trials. It appears useful to have a closer look at studies with fluoxetine and escitalopram which were outstanding from the rest of the paediatric antidepressant trials. First a short summary of two major paediatric *fluoxetine* studies is provided which showed efficacy in paediatric (both children and adolescents) populations. The first (Emslie et al., 1997) had two treatment arms (fluoxetine and placebo), and only 48 subjects were allocated to each of these arms (for comparison, the median sample size per treatment arm for the studies reviewed by Bridge et al. (2009) was 110 subjects). In spite of the relatively low sample size, there was a statistically significant difference between fluoxetine and placebo on the CDRS-R total score (Children's Depression Rating Scale, Revised: Poznanski and Mokros, 1996) (last observation carried forward analysis). The responder rates (based on CGI-I categories) were 56% for fluoxetine (20 mg) and 33% for placebo ($\Delta = 23\%$) – which is a fairly good separation of treatment effects, when compared with the average approximately 13% reported by Bridge et al. (2009). There were no differences in response rates between children and adolescent subgroup. The second fluoxetine study (Emslie et al., 2002) was conducted at 15 sites in the United States and comprised a total of 219 randomised MDD patients (122 children and 97 adolescents) treated for 8 weeks with either fluoxetine 20 mg or placebo. Again, fluoxetine was significantly superior to placebo on the CDRS-R total score (Poznanski and Mokros, 1996) ($P < .001$), on the Montgomery–Asberg Depression Rating Scale (Montgomery and Asberg, 1979) ($P = .023$) and the Clinical Global Impression of Severity Scale (Guy, 1976). The responder rate analysis, based on a changes from baseline of at least 30% in the CDRS-R total score, showed 65% responders under fluoxetine and 53% under placebo (i.e. $\Delta = 12\%$).

The first *escitalopram* study (Wagner et al., 2006), which was part of Bridge et al. (2009) meta-analysis, included children and adolescents (6–17 years) with MDD. These were randomised to an 8-week treatment with either 10–20 mg escitalopram ($n = 131$) or placebo ($n = 133$). There was no statistically significant treatment difference on the primary outcome measure, the CDRS-R total score (least-squares mean difference was -1.7; $P = .31$). However, in post hoc analyses, escitalopram was significantly superior to placebo in the group of adolescents (least-squares mean difference of -4.6, $P = .47$) but not in children. This post hoc finding was confirmed by a second study that included adolescent subjects (12–17 years of age) only (Emslie et al., 2009).

The overall picture of success rates of antidepressant studies in paediatric MDD, summarised so far (for the years 1966–2009), has not changed in more recent studies. A recent major international program with duloxetine in MDD was conducted between 2009 and 2011 in children (7–11 years) and adolescents (12–17 years). It consisted of two major international phase 3 studies. Duloxetine is a newer antidepressant, a dual serotonin–norepinephrine reuptake inhibitor (SNRI), which has gained worldwide market approval for the treatment of adult MDD in 2004. Doses selected for the two paediatric phase 3 trials were carefully tested in a paediatric phase 2 pharmacokinetic and tolerance study (Prakash et al., 2012). In both phase 3 efficacy and tolerance studies, approximately 59% of the subjects were adolescents and 41% children. Females and males were almost equally represented. Both studies compared duloxetine with placebo and fluoxetine (active comparator) in a 10-week acute treatment duration, using a double-blind, randomised group design. The study design of both studies was similar with the exception of the number of treatment arms and dosing (flexible dosing vs fixed doses). The studies were conducted in different geographical regions. The *first* study (Emslie et al., 2014) included 60 study sites, distributed over the United States, Canada, Mexico, and Argentina, used fixed doses of the study drugs and comprised 463 subjects randomised (1:1:1:1) to four treatment arms of acute treatment (1) duloxetine 60 mg QD, (2) duloxetine 30 mg QD, (3) fluoxetine 20 mg QD, and (4) placebo. The *second* study (Atkinson et al., 2014) used 65 study sites, that were distributed over Europe (Estonia, Finland, France, Germany, Slovakia, Russia, and Ukraine), South Africa, and the United States, and comprised 337 randomised patients allocated (1:1:1) to three treatment arms with flexible dosing ((1) duloxetine (60–120 mg QD), (2) fluoxetine (20–40 mg QD, and (3) placebo). A particular feature of these studies, which makes them distinct from all other paediatric MDD studies reviewed earlier, was that they used, besides placebo, fluoxetine as an active comparator, that is, the only drug that has received regulatory approval for the treatment of children and adolescents with MDD. Both studies showed consistent but disappointing efficacy results. Neither duloxetine nor fluoxetine was significantly different from placebo on the primary outcome variable (CDRS-R total score). This is reflected in the response rates (defined as >50% improvement on CDRS-R total score from baseline):

- response rates in study 1 (60 sites in the United States, Canada, Mexico, and Argentina) (Emslie et al., 2014)
  - for duloxetine 60 mg QD: 69%
  - for duloxetine 30 mg QD: 69%
  - for fluoxetine 20 mg QD: 61%
  - for placebo: 61%
  - Δ (best active drug rates vs placebo) 8%
- response rates in study 2 (65 sites in various European countries, South Africa, and the United States) (Atkinson et al., 2014)
  - for duloxetine (60–120 mg QD): 67%
  - for fluoxetine (20–40 mg QD): 63%
  - for placebo: 62%
  - Δ (best active drug rates vs placebo) 5%

The most remarkable finding of these studies was that even the antidepressant standard with established efficacy in paediatric populations (fluoxetine) could not be separated from placebo. This allows the firm conclusion that these studies were indeed failed (false-negative) trials.

The overall conclusion from the earlier review of paediatric MDD studies is that, over the last 50 years (1966 until today), approximately 15 (or more) antidepressant drugs have been tested in double-blind, placebo-controlled studies in children and adolescents with MDD. Almost all of these clinical trials, with the exception of a few fluoxetine and escitalopram studies, failed to demonstrate superiority over placebo. Even the positive findings with fluoxetine could not be replicated in the recent duloxetine studies. Both adult and paediatric MDD studies share the common issue of indiscriminative trials and high placebo response rates. Whereas the study failure rate in adults is about 50%, it appears to be 90% and higher in paediatric studies. Unfortunately, this situation has not improved over time, as the most recent duloxetine studies show. In the contrary, reviews and metaanalyses, comparing older with more recently conducted antidepressant efficacy trials in MDD, have detected trends of increased placebo response rates over time which appear to be similar for adult and paediatric studies. For studies in *adult MDD*, Walsh et al. (2002) found a significant increase in responder rates over approximately 20 years (1981–2000), with a markedly stronger trend for *placebo* response ($r=0.45$, $P<.001$) than for response under *active drug* treatment ($r=0.26$, $P=.02$). In a recent publication (Khan et al., 2017), which comprised all adult studies with antidepressants in MDD submitted to the FDA from 1985 to 2015, that is, over 30 years, these trends could be confirmed: the correlation coefficients (response rates vs time of submission) were $r=0.46$ ($P<.001$) for placebo responders and 0.37 ($P<.001$) for responders under active drugs. A similar trend of an increasing number of *placebo r*esponders over time (between 1997 and 2007) was reported by Bridge et al. (2009) for paediatric depression trials. The year of publication of these studies was significantly correlated with the proportion of *placebo* responders ($r=0.64$, $P=.05$), that is, more recently published studies reported higher placebo response rates than older publications. Further analyses of this relationship identified two main factors accounting for this temporal trend (Bridge et al., 2009): (a) a 'publication artifact' and (b) an increasing number of study sites involved in these studies over time ($r = 0.69$; $P = .03$). The 'publication artifact' was related to differences in time lag between study completion and year of publication. Whereas positive studies were published within 2 years, it took about almost 5 years to publish failed studies. A further confirmation of the trend of increased placebo response in paediatric MDD studies over time comes from a comparison of placebo response rates (averages for children and adolescents) provided by Bridge et al. (2009) (covering published studies from 1988 to 2006) and Cohen et al. (2008) (covering studies from 1972 to 2007), with the recent figures from the duloxetine paediatric program:

- placebo response rates according to Cohen et al. (2008): 49.6%
- placebo response rates according to Bridge et al. (2009): 46.0%
- placebo response rates found in the two duloxetine studies (Emslie et al., 2014; Atkinson et al., 2014): 61% and 62%

9.4 Magnitude and range of placebo response in adult and paediatric populations with different mental disorders

The previous section described the magnitude and scope of placebo effects and study failures for trials with antidepressants in MDD. This section will address the question whether these findings are specific, perhaps even exceptional for MDD studies, or can be generalised to other mental disorders. Its objective is to investigate if there are any systematic variations in placebo response across different mental disorders and age populations. Specifically, it will be attempted to answer the following two questions:

(1) Are there *systematic differences* in the magnitude and range of *placebo response* rates *between paediatric mental disorders*?
(2) Are there patterns of systematic *age-associated differences* (i.e. between children, adolescents, and adults) in placebo response rates?

Cohen et al. (2008) undertook a Medline database search for publications on randomised, placebo-controlled, parallel-group medication trials in *children and adolescents with major depression (MDD), obsessive–compulsive disorder (OCD), and other 'non-OCD anxiety disorders'*. They found 70 studies published between January 1972 and October 2007, and 40 of these met all of their selection criteria (including blinding procedures, randomisation, parallel-group design, sufficient information on inclusion/ exclusion criteria, treatment, responder definitions, and evaluations). Twenty-three of these studies (57.5%) were MDD trials, 7 OCD (17.5%), and 10 (non-OCD) anxiety disorder trials (25%). A total of 2533 patients were on active drug and 1528 on placebo. Metaanalyses with the pooled data provided the following results:

- *differences in the magnitude and range of placebo response rates between paediatric mental disorders*

Placebo response rate were significantly higher for MDD than for OCD and other anxiety disorders ($P = .002$):
- MDD: 49.6% (range: 17%–90%)
- OCD: 31% (range: 4%–41%)
- anxiety disorders (non-OCD): 39.6% (range: 9%–53%)

Since the earlier metaanalysis only included depressive and anxiety disorders, additional literature can help to supplement the earlier information with placebo response rates for other paediatric mental disorders:
- attention deficit hyperactivity disorder (ADHD) (children only) about 30% (Parellada et al., 2012; Sandler et al., 2008)
- schizophrenia (adolescents) 26%–36% (Haas et al., 2009; Parellada et al., 2012).

- *differences in placebo response between age groups (Table 9.1)*

  A. *Within the paediatric population, that is, comparison of children vs adolescents*

  Only a subgroup of the studies (composed of 567 children and 1171 adolescents), reviewed by Cohen et al. (2008), provided relevant information on differences in placebo response between children and adolescents. Although these differences did not reach the level of statistical significance ($t = 1.12$; $P = .27$), their direction was consistent across the diagnostic groups, suggesting systematic trends rather than random variations. Placebo response rates in
  - MDD: 60% in children versus 49% in adolescents[a]
  - OCD: 40% in children versus 32% in adolescents
  - anxiety disorders: 42% in children versus 32% in adolescents

  B. *Adult placebo response rates*

  For *adult patients* the following *placebo response rates* were provided by Weimer et al. (2013, referencing Fineberg et al., 2006; Rutherford et al., 2009; Stein et al., 2006; Wilens et al., 2002):
  - MDD: 38%
  - OCD: 33%
  - ADHD: 10%

  For schizophrenia trials the average placebo responder rate *in adults* was estimated to be 25% (range: 0%–41%) (Kinon et al., 2011), whereas the placebo responder rates for *children* was in the range of 26%–36% (Parellada et al., 2012).

Table 9.1 Reported placebo response rates in paediatric populations and adults (see text for references).

Type of disorder	Placebo responders		
	Children (%)	Adolescents (%)	Adults (%)
MDD	60	49	38
OCD	40	32	33
Anxiety disorders	42	32	–
Schizophrenia	26–36	–	25

[a] Bridge et al. (2009) provided in their review the following placebo response rates for MDD: 49.6% in children and 44.5% in adolescents.

The earlier overview of findings provides a fairly consistent picture that allows to address the questions raised at the beginning of this section:

(1) In all of the mental disorders for which sufficient information was available from both paediatric and adult studies, *substantial placebo response rates* were found. This includes major depressive disorder (MDD), anxiety disorders, obsessive–compulsive disorder (OCS), attention deficit hyperactivity (ADHD), and schizophrenia. Considering information from adult studies on other mental disorders, not included in the earlier list, substantial placebo response rates can be expected for (almost) all types of mental disorders both in adult and paediatric populations.
(2) There are consistent differences in the magnitude of placebo effects *between the different types of mental disorders*. Depressive disorders show the highest placebo responder rates, followed by anxiety disorders, OCD, schizophrenia, and ADHD. This suggests that the disease/disorder type is an important moderator of placebo effects.
(3) In the patient populations analyzed, *consistent differences in the magnitude of placebo responder rates were found between different age populations*, with children showing the highest, adolescents intermediate, and adults the lowest placebo responder rates.

Based upon these conclusions, one would expect a particularly high risk of study failure (false-negative studies due to high placebo response rates) for studies in paediatric depression and anxiety disorders and lower risks for ADHD studies. Overall, there is a monotonous trend of an increasing risk of study failure due to placebo response rates from older to younger populations, with children studies associated with the highest risk and adult studies with the lowest, though still significant risk.

9.5 Factors of placebo effects

Any proposal of effective measures that can reduce the risk of increased placebo effects requires a good understanding of the factors driving and facilitating these effects. This section will provide an overview of findings and hypotheses on factors and processes that are likely to cause and facilitate placebo effects. It will be important to separate the factors for 'perceived' and 'true' effects.

9.5.1 Factors of 'perceived' (artificial) placebo effects

There are multiple reasons for 'perceived' or artificial placebo response, and these can be driven by unintentional or deliberate, intentional strategies:

- The *tendency of patients to report a more favourable therapeutic outcome*
  This type of selective, biased reporting of therapeutic results is sometimes described in the therapeutic literature as a 'hello–goodbye effect' (Choi and Pak, 2007). It refers to the tendency of patients to exaggerate their problems before a treatment (in order to receive the necessary help) and to minimise them and exaggerate improvements at the end (out of gratitude and/or to please the therapist). Another possible explanation of this tendency is offered by Festinger's (1957) theory of 'cognitive dissonance': Individuals strive towards consistency within themselves, and inconsistencies ('dissonance') between beliefs and the perception of one's own actions are experienced as unpleasant. An example of such inconsistencies could be the perceived 'investments' into a therapy or therapeutic study

(e.g. efforts to regularly visit the therapist, travel to the study site, and undergo frequent, lengthy assessments), on one hand, and a disappointing therapeutic outcome, on the other. One way to resolve this 'dissonance' is to change one's beliefs/evaluation of the outcome of the therapy, that is, to consider it as more favourable than it was.

- *Other rater biases,* such as the tendency in observer ratings, called *'generosity'* (Cronbach, 1970, p. 572)

  Whereas the hello–goodbye effect is shaping patient reports, this tendency is affecting investigators. It is a tendency to give favourable reports as a reflection of a therapist's or investigator's beliefs in his own therapeutic experience and skills. It could be also a reflection of the investigators' favourable attitude towards the investigational product.

- *A phenomenon called 'baseline score inflation'*

  A tendency of clinical investigators to increase patients' baseline severity scores so that they reach the minimal severity level defined in the study protocol and make patients eligible for the study. This tendency is elicited and reinforced by recruitment pressure and by financial incentives. Studies have shown that, after patients are finally enrolled into a clinical trial, score inflation tendencies in postbaseline ratings tend to decrease or disappear. This creates artificial (or 'perceived') endpoint-baseline differences suggestive of an improvement. Evidence for baseline score inflations comes from studies that used additional measures of symptom severity independent from investigators ratings, either patient self-ratings or ratings from other raters, for example, central ratings (Byrom and Mundt, 2005; Landin et al., 2000).

- *'Regression to the mean'* as another possible source of 'perceived' placebo effects (Bland and Altman, 1994)

  This is a statistical phenomenon associated to random errors in repeated measurements. Assessments are associated with measurement errors due to the relative unreliability of measures (e.g. scale assessments). These errors are assumed to show a normal (Gaussian) distribution around the 'true' value of a variable, estimated by the mean of all possible measures. In repeated measures, initially extreme values tend to normalise, that is, regress to the mean ('true value') of the distribution. Specifically, initial values suggesting extremely severe levels of symptom expression would be likely to be reduced (i.e. indicative of a reduction in severity) in repeated assessments and thus create an artificial placebo effect. The amount of contribution of this statistical phenomenon to the issue of placebo effects in clinical trials is unclear. Theoretically, regression to the mean could occur with extreme values on both ends, not only with extremely high but also with extremely low baseline severity values. The latter would create artificial worsening. This would correct for the artificial placebo effect when calculating mean efficacy values per treatment group. However, in clinical studies, artificial worsening may occur less frequently because study protocols restrict the inclusion of very mildly ill patients by defining a minimum severity score.

9.5.2 Factors of 'true' placebo effects

Reviews of studies dealing with factors and sources of 'true' placebo effects and discussions of their possible relevance for paediatric psychopharmacology have been provided by various recent publications (e.g. Parellada et al., 2012; Rutherford and Roose, 2013; Simmons et al., 2014; Weimer et al., 2013). The majority of these studies come from trials conducted in a few disease/disorder areas (mainly depression and pain). In the succeeding text, it will be attempted to integrate and summarise the factors of 'true' placebo effects by suggesting a general model of placebo effects. Conclusions on factors of placebo response are usually based on retrospective ('posthoc') analyses, and there are only a few factors for which findings were replicated (e.g. the influence of disease severity on placebo effects). Therefore any suggestion of *a general model of placebo effects, in particular for paediatric psychopharmacology,* is necessarily based on a mixture of a few relatively solid findings and an array of plausible hypothetical factors for which only some degree of evidence is available. In spite of these limitations, such a model appears to have several important merits. It enables an integration of scattered findings and assumptions into a relatively consistent context, suggests possible interactions of the factors of placebo effects, and puts them in a temporal order of more distant versus more immediate conditions. This will be important for recommendations of measures for the reduction of placebo effects because remote influences and conditions in the past are hard to change. Another advantage of such a model is its heuristic (hypothesis-creating) value for future research on factors and sources of placebo effects.

'True' placebo effects, that is, real improvements of patients' clinical condition due to psychological effects arising in the psychosocial context of therapeutic settings, have been shown to have *neurobiological correlates.* Evidence suggests that the pattern of the neurobiological mechanisms is determined by two major components: (a) a disorder-specific component, changes or processes associated with the improvement of the specific type of disorder/disease in question, and (b) a disease-independent component, changes that are likely to reflect the contribution of reward (or 'improvement') expectation (Benedetti et al., 2005; Mayberg et al., 2002). The disease-specific neurobiological changes are similar (but not identical) to those observed under active treatment (drug treatment or psychotherapy) of the specific type of disorder (e.g. depression). For example, for depression treatment, positron emission tomography (PET) investigations and regional cerebral blood flow studies have shown changes in cortical areas and limbic-/paralimbic-cortical circuits known to be implicated in emotion and stress regulation and in the pathophysiology of depression. These include the anterior cingulate cortex, the insula, nucleus accumbens, and subcortical regions (caudate, thalamus, and brain stem) (Benedetti et al., 2005; Pecina et al., 2015). Whereas changes in frontal regions have been observed in all types of depression treatment, other regional brain effects seemed to vary with the specific type of treatment (i.e. antidepressant drug treatment vs specific psychotherapeutic interventions). The disease-independent effects, presumably associated to placebo-specific processes, involve changes in the ventral striatum and orbital frontal cortex. These are processes typically observed in the expectation and delivery of reward in conditioned learning experiments (Benedetti et al., 2005).

Neurobiological findings and models give particular credibility to the notion that placebo effects reflect true, real changes, and they enhance our understanding of their powerful nature. But they cannot replace psychological models, that is, models that link placebo effects to specific types of experiences and behaviours that occur in therapeutic settings. The identification of these types of experiences and behaviours, by which placebo effects are elicited, is the prerequisite of any recommendations on how to avoid or reduce placebo effects in clinical efficacy studies (Geers and Miller, 2014). Two major theories have been proposed to account for processes generating placebo effects in the psychosocial context of therapeutic settings, (a) *the (cognitive) expectancy theory* (i.e. expectations of health improvement) and (b) the *classical (Pavlovian) conditioning theory of placebo effects* (Geers and Miller, 2014; Stewart-Williams and Podd, 2004). Both theories have often been presented as competitive alternatives, the first focusing on *conscious* processes based on verbal information and the second relating to *nonconscious* processes describing the acquisition of placebo effects as a result of stimulus–stimulus conditioning in former similar therapeutic settings. However, both appear to offer rather complementary than mutually excluding explanations. First, modern cognitive theories and models, based on information-processing paradigms, do not require fully conscious processes for the generation of expectation. They may involve automatic (nonconscious) and partly and fully explicit (conscious) processes. Phenomenological investigations of health improvement expectations occurring in therapeutic settings are likely to show a big variability of processes that range from fully consciously elaborated thoughts and feelings, that can be easily verbalised, to diffuse and vague anticipatory 'feelings'. Second the information used for the creation of health expectations does not only come from (explicit) verbal communications but from gestures, mimics, emotional undertones of statements, and patients' observations of the investigator. Third, classical conditioning theory may better explain the association between specific physiological and immunological processes and the therapeutic setting, whereas expectancy theory seems to make better understanding of the influence of verbally transmitted information about a treatment in a therapeutic setting. The formation of health improvement expectations can involve various types of learning processes, not only classical conditioning and (conscious) verbal learning but also operant conditioning (by 'social reinforcement'), incidental (implicit) learning, and imitation learning based on the observation of the behaviour and attitudes of models (usually represented by so-called significant others) (Bandura, 1971; Kirsch, 1997; Montgomery and Kirsch, 1997; Rachman, 1977; Stewart-Williams and Podd, 2004). According to schema theories (Beck et al., 1979; Eysenck and Keane, 2010), expectations are based on 'schemata', which are specific long-term memory structures that reflect the integration of sediments (or 'traces') of former experience and acquired knowledge about specific classes of events. These schemata tend to filter and shape the acquisition (attention, perception, interpretation, and encoding) of new relevant information in specific settings, its storage and consolidation and its recall in similar future settings. They also determine the type of emotions associated with these cognitions.

Some researchers (Rutherford and Roose, 2013; Rutherford et al., 2011) raise doubts in the *explanatory value of the expectancy theory of placebo effects*. They argue that the fact that children show the highest rates of placebo response speaks against the expectancy theory because children have a limited (cognitive) capacity of understanding (verbal) information on clinical trials (e.g. provided in information for informed consent and assent). The expectancy theory would therefore falsely predict a stronger placebo effect in adults because of their capacity to better understand and elaborate verbal information. This argument is based on the misunderstanding that expectations need to be fully consciously elaborated and based on verbal information learning only or mainly. The authors are correct in pointing out the relative modest explanatory power of a pure expectancy theory of placebo effects and by emphasizing the particular importance of the therapeutic setting. One needs, however, to distinguish between immediate processes mediating and determining placebo effects (i.e. the development of specific expectations of health improvement) and their antecedent causes and conditions (i.e. the context eliciting them). Expectations (here, health improvement expectations) seem to be key as modulators of placebo effects, but the likelihood of their occurrence and their strength and quality will be dependent on antecedent factors and conditions among which the nature of the therapeutic setting appears to be prominent but not the only immediate sources of placebo effects.

The following factors and conditions and their interactions are suggested to be predictors of health improvement expectations that are underlying ('true') placebo effects and determine their occurrence, magnitude, and frequency.

The following will explain the features of placebo effects summarised in Table 9.2 and provide some further explanations:

(i) *Predisposing factors as moderator variables of the strength of health improvement expectations ('risk or "vulnerability" factors for placebo effects' – Group 1 of 'distal' antecedent factors)*
   a. Current disease characteristics
   Type of disease/disorder, disease severity, disease complexity (i.e. with or without co-morbidities), disease chronicity, and natural course of disease (e.g. progressive or phasic with spontaneous remissions). Note: See previous section for figures on differences in placebo effects between different mental diseases/disorders. Disease severity as a factor of placebo response is one of the best replicated findings (Khan et al., 2002, 2005; Kirsch, 2008).

Table 9.2 Features of a (hypothetical) model of 'true' placebo effects (overview).

Factor type	Factor subgroups
1. Predisposing (or 'risk') factors	Current disease characteristics, age, gender, developmental status, specific personality traits, degree of suggestibility, history of own, and significant others' health problems
2. Social environment factors (supporting health improvement expectations)	Attitudes of significant others towards physicians/health care professionals, clinical trials; expectations of significant others regarding treatment outcome, including health anxiety of significant others; reputation/prestige of medical institution and team
3. Acute ('proximal') situational factors – the therapeutic setting	Information on study/study treatment received by medical staff, clinicians' attitudes (towards patient) and clinicians' personality traits, clinicians' remarks and (possible) psychotherapeutic actions, emotional quality of patient–clinician interaction, length and frequency of patient–clinician interaction
4. Acute health improvement expectations mediating placebo response	Patients' acute perception of their own health problem, their acute health-related anxiety, retrieved experience with health problems, perceived medical competence and trustworthiness of clinician(s)/investigator(s), interpretation of study information provided. Strength of health improvement expectation

b. Age, gender, and developmental status (neurobiological, cognitive, and emotional)
Data presented in previous sections of this article clearly support the influence of age (children vs adolescents vs adults) on the magnitude and frequency of placebo response (for 'developmental status', see comments further in the succeeding text).
c. Specific personality traits
The following traits and relatively enduring personal characteristics have been proposed in the literature: strength of trait anxiety and neuroticism, extraversion/ introversion (especially, sociability and trustfulness in social situations), coping skills, and general outcome expectancies (associated with the degree of self-esteem, specific self-concepts of mental and physical health, (perceived) locus of control and self-efficiency to handle problems, and dispositional optimism vs pessimism) (Bandura, 1997; Geers et al., 2010; Reynaert et al., 1995; Rutherford and Roose, 2013; Weimer et al., 2013).
d. Degree of suggestibility
That is the susceptibility to be influenced in social interactions by others (their opinions and attitudes), especially persons with authority or 'significant others' (i.e. parents, other relatives, partners, and friends) (De Pascalis et al., 2002; Parellada et al., 2012; Simmons et al., 2014; Weimer et al., 2013).
e. History of own and significant others' health problems and their outcome

(ii) *Social environment factors shaping and supporting health improvement expectations (Group 2 of 'distal' antecedent factors)*
a. Attitudes of 'significant others' towards physicians and health care professionals
b. Attitudes of 'significant others' towards clinical studies and medical research (i.e. their value, risks, and possible benefits)
c. Treatment outcome expectations of 'significant others' regarding medical treatment in general and treatment of the specific disease in question in specific
d. Type of coping behaviour with health problems, promoted by 'significant others' (Simmons et al., 2014; Vervoort et al., 2011)
e. Anxiety, specifically health-related anxiety of 'significant others' (Simmons et al., 2014)
f. Reputation and prestige of the medical institution and medical team

(iii) *Situational factors eliciting health improvement expectations and behavioural change ('immediate', 'proximal', or 'acute' antecedents and eliciting factors of health improvement expectations and behavioural changes)*
a. Type of information on (study) treatment provided by study personnel/medical staff
Specifically a balanced or unbalanced description of possible risks and benefits, the chance of receiving a placebo drug, verbal code, and complexity of information presented (relative to individual's cognitive complexity level).
b. Factors of the therapeutic setting – clinician's attitudes and personality
Clinicians' attitudes towards the patients in the clinician–patient interaction and his/her personality determine the strength and quality of the therapeutic bond or alliance (Rutherford and Roose, 2013; Simmons et al., 2014). Attitudes and behaviour facilitating a strong and good relationship include his/her affective attitude, especially emotional warms, empathy, and experiential congruence (i.e. the consistency of his/her shown behaviour and statements with his/her true attitudes and thoughts inferred by the patient). The latter determines the investigator's/therapist's trustworthiness, as perceived by the patient. These types of behaviour were suggested by Rogers (1957), the founder of client-centered therapy, as essential for a successful psychotherapy. They were also identified in so-called generic ('school-independent') models of psychotherapy as basic

factors and facilitators of therapeutic change (Orlinsky and Howard, 1987; Orlinsky et al., 2004).

c. Factors of the therapeutic setting – types of clinicians' remarks, comments, and behaviour with potential psychotherapeutic influence

In an attempt to help their patients, clinicians/investigators and medical staff may not only spontaneously and incidentally but also deliberately provide some degree of counselling to their patients, using techniques similar to those known from formal counselling and psychotherapies. Examples are advice on stress and time management and activity plans; remarks on patients' attitudes and dysfunctional beliefs (e.g. regarding their health problems); comments on specific coping skills, reminding them of their abilities and strengths (i.e. in an attempt to activate possible 'therapeutic resources') and helping them to structure and better understand their conflicts; and remarks on the efficacy of the administered medication. (Examples: 'I am sure your problem will improve over the next few weeks'. 'You are making progress'.). Such reinsuring remarks are often provoked by direct questions of the patient ('Am I making progress?').

d. Length and frequency of investigator/medical staff and patient interactions (both per visit day and the length of intervals between visit days)

Longer and more frequent interactions are likely to enhance the chances of the development of good, emotionally rewarding patient–investigator interactions (Posternak and Zimmerman, 2007; Robinson and Rickels, 2000; Rutherford and Roose, 2013). Typical examples are lengthy assessment periods (interviews and clinical scale administrations) on visit days and frequent assessment days within short intervals.

(iv) *Factors and features of the acute health improvement expectations mediating placebo effects*

a. Patient's perceived (own) health problem (his/her subjective focus, its perceived features, quality, severity, and seriousness)
b. Patient's (degree of) acute health-related anxiety
c. Patient's (retrieved) memories of own and 'significant others' experience with health problems (e.g. degree and speed of improvement and recovery)
d. Patient's perception of the medical 'competence' of the investigator/medical staff
e. Patient's understanding, interpretation of information received on treatment and study procedures, his/her emotional reactions, and his/her evaluation of the reliability and trustworthiness of this information

The developing health improvement expectation(s) will produce selective attention, filtering and weighing of received information that is consistent with the expectations. These trigger top-down mechanisms in the brain that influence the areas and neural circuits related to the symptoms in question.

Which factors of the outlined model of placebo effects are likely to account for the marked differences in magnitude and frequency of placebo effects between children, adolescents, and adults? Why do children tend to have stronger placebo effects than adolescents and adults?

Table 9.3 suggests that differences in the magnitude of placebo effects are mainly determined by three related factor groups: the *developmental status*, the *'suggestibility'* of children versus adolescents and adults, and the quality and strength of the *patient–investigator/clinician relationship* (Parellada et al., 2012; Rutherford and Roose, 2013; Simmons et al., 2014; Weimer et al., 2013). 'Differences in developmental status comprise the neurobiological development and the related status of cognitive and emotional functions. These account for differences in disease concepts (i.e. the perceived nature

Table 9.3 Factors likely to account for differences in 'true' placebo effects between children, adolescents, and adults.

Differentiating factor	Factor description
Developmental status	Neurobiological developmental status and cognitive and emotional developmental status
Strength/degree of suggestibility	Increased suggestibility in children, compared with adolescents and adults; enhanced preparedness and susceptibility to be influenced by (trustworthy) models/authority figures
Quality and strength of patient–clinician interaction	In children more intense emotional interactions with clinician(s)

and complexity of their current disease/disorder, the factors causing and controlling it, and the more 'subjective' nature of these concepts) (Seiffge-Krenke, 2008), the (perceived) 'locus of control' and children's 'dispositional optimism' (Geers et al., 2010; Weimer et al., 2013), and capabilities of emotion regulation (Holodynski and Oerter, 2008). Compared with adults and adolescents, children are likely to have less complex and neutral ('objective') concepts of their disease, and these tend to be more influenced by emotions (e.g. anxiety) than in adults. It is easier for children, compared with adolescents and adults, to ignore problems and show 'optimism' (belief of improvement), partly even associated with 'magical thinking', provided a trustful and competent person (e.g. the clinician/investigator) gives reasons for such optimism. Increased 'suggestibility', that is, an enhanced preparedness or susceptibility to be influenced by models and authority figures (such as clinicians and 'significant others'), seems to be a reflection of children's developmental status. In a review of the literature on differences in suggestibility, Parellada et al. (2012) suggest that about 15% of the adult population are 'highly suggestible', compared with 80% of children with approximately 12 years of age (De Pascalis et al., 2002; Page and Green, 2007). Suggestibility is triggered by specific situations of social interaction which involve an identification with models. The likelihood of interaction partners to become models is increased by the following properties: promise of emotional support, competence, social status, and power over gratifying resources (Bandura, 1971). 'Good clinicians' are perceived by their patients to have several of these properties (see the earlier general model of placebo effects for behaviour and attitudes of therapists facilitating therapeutic change). The increased suggestibility of children is therefore to be considered as a characteristic feature of their more intense therapeutic relationship with their clinicians/investigators and their staff. The increased suggestibility of children and their preparedness to engage in emotional interactions with 'models' represent natural developmental conditions to facilitate social learning and the acquisition of social and emotional skills, including techniques of coping with stress and emotion regulation in difficult situations. Children's enhanced suggestibility and preparedness to engage in emotional interactions with models explain also the nature of their expectations (including health improvement expectations). These tend to be strongly influenced by emotional undertones of the therapeutic relationship and more by connotations than the denotations of verbal messages.

An important factor of the quality and strength of the child–clinician relationship is likely to be the quality of parent–clinician interactions, as perceived by the child (Tates and Meeuwesen, 2001; Simmons et al., 2014).

9.5.3 Increased variability of outcome measures as a source of indiscriminative (false-negative) efficacy studies

In a previous section of this article, it was pointed out that enhanced placebo effects represent only one, though an important source of indiscriminative (false-negative) studies. Another important source is the enhanced variability of outcome measures (Kobak et al., 2007). More precisely, this issue is caused by unexpectedly large within-(treatment) group variances, in comparison with the between-group variances. The larger the variances of the primary outcome measure *within* the treatment groups (intragroup variances), compared with the variance(s) *between* the treatment groups (intergroup variances), the more likely the study will be indiscriminative, that is, cannot differentiate between active drug and placebo effects.

For a further analysis of this issue, one needs to consider the basic assumptions ('axioms') and the reliability concept of classical measurement (or test) theory (Fischer, 1974; Gulliksen, 1950). According to this theory an *observed value* of a variable (e.g. a scale score or value of another type of outcome measure) consists of two (additive) components, a *'true' value* and a *'measurement error' value*. The latter determines the reliability of the measure. The greater the measurement error, the lower the reliability of the assessment. Accordingly the reasons for large intra-(treatment) group variances could be large 'true' variances or large 'error variances' or both. 'True' outcome measure variances reflect the (true) *heterogeneity of response of the patient sample*. Changes in patient selection criteria that result in more homogeneous patient groups could help to reduce this variance component. But such changes need to be carefully considered. First, one would ideally need to know which patient characteristics determine treatment response. This is often not known. Secondly, attempts to reduce the response variances by reducing the heterogeneity of the used patient sample could raise concerns about the representativity of the patient sample and the generalizability of the study results to existing diagnostic categories. Such concerns can lead to difficult discussions with regulatory authorities about the labelling of the new drug (i.e. the specification of its 'indication'). Therefore, before considering a reduction of the 'true' variance of outcome measures, it appears advisable to first try to *reduce the error variance of the primary outcome measure*. The following factors of error variances need to be considered:

- The unreliability of the used clinical scale and assessments
    Relative low interrater reliabilities are due to variations in patient assessments, for example, by semi- or unstructured interviews and insufficiently defined scoring rules. The impact of low interrater reliabilities is further enhanced by large numbers of study sites and the inclusion of sites from many countries with different languages and cultures, sites with low numbers of patients (especially with numbers lower than two or three times the number of treatment arms used in the study), and frequent changes of raters and in the sequence of scale administrations. Large systematic differences in findings between study sites could even

lead to significant treatment–centre interactions (i.e. different signals coming from different study sites) that can make the study results uninterpretable.
- Study conduct problems due to protocol violations
  The higher the frequency of violations, the bigger the influence of these problems on the size of the error variance.
- Deviations from protocol specifications due to the allowance of protocol waivers (for patient entry criteria or prohibited concomitant medication) – with the possible consequence of less control of confounding influences on treatment effects.

9.6 Measures to reduce the number of indiscriminative (false-negative) efficacy studies in paediatric psychopharmacology

Considering the multiple factors of indiscriminative (false-negative) studies discussed earlier, a single measure will not markedly change the magnitude of this issue. Attempts to *influence the quality of clinician/investigator–patient interactions and control the development of strong health improvement expectations* are useful but may have limited success, especially in paediatric populations. The usual recommendations involve the following: Clinical investigators need to show a neutral, research-oriented attitude in their interactions with patients and provide balanced information on the risks and possible benefits of the investigated treatment, in particular on the possibility that patients may receive a placebo drug. They should avoid any specific statements that are likely to influence and reinforce patients' treatment expectations. They should not make use of measures with possible therapeutic effects, such as those borrowed from counselling or quasitherapeutic techniques. Reminding investigators (and their staff) of these factors needs to be an obligatory part of an investigators' training. The limitations of these attempts, especially when dealing with paediatric populations, are the following: First, it will be difficult, even for experienced investigators, to control their own behaviour and interactions with patients because they cannot change their own temperamental traits. In such interactions, a major part of behavioural reactions will be automatically elicited and be not or only partially under conscious control. Second, considering the discussed features of the developmental status of children and adolescents, neutral, strongly controlled investigators' behaviour may not have neutral but negative effects on patients' willingness to cooperate and on their treatment compliance. There is a fine line between a research-oriented neutrality and a negative impact on the therapeutic alliance. Third the impact of verbal information, which describes the risks and benefits of a treatment in a balanced way, is limited in children and, though generally to a lesser degree, in adolescents. Due to their developmental status and their increased suggestibility, they show an enhanced proneness to emotional cues and other non-verbal information provided in the investigator/clinician–patient interaction. For the earlier reasons, it may be difficult to influence the quality of the patient–clinician interaction, but the length and frequency of such interactions could be controlled by avoiding lengthy and frequent assessments.

In view of these limitations of attempts to influence the investigator/patient relationship, approaches to *reduce artificial ('perceived') placebo effects* are likely to have a higher probability of success. This applies to the effects of baseline score inflations and *the (intragroup) variance of outcome measures*. Attempts to reduce the occurrence of baseline score inflations have successfully used a combination of the following strategies: blinding raters at individual study sites to the timing of baseline assessments and randomisation, using separate clinical scales for patients' eligibility to the study (i.e. severity of the disease) and baseline assessment (e.g. two different clinician rating scales or a clinician-rated and a patient-rated scale), and using centralised ratings (Byrom and Mundt, 2005; Rutherford and Roose, 2013).

Another approach to reduce the risk of false-negative trials would be strategies to *reduce the size of 'true' intragroup variances of outcome* measures by so-called enrichment strategies for clinical trials (Food and Drug Administration (FDA), 2012). These try to increase the discriminatory power of a clinical trial by either selecting patients with more homogeneous therapeutic effects or excluding patients that are likely to increase the variance of these effects. A prerequisite of strategies of 'prognostic enrichment' is the a priori identification of valid response predictors. An example would be a patient selection based on disease severity. Indeed, given the inverse relationship between severity of disease and the magnitude of placebo effect, it is recommendable to exclude patients with a mild severity of a mental disorder from an efficacy study. However, with the exception of the factor 'disease severity', knowledge of powerful response predictors is rarely available in clinical psychopharmacology which is why researchers mainly try to make use of so-called empiric selection strategies (FDA, 2012). Examples of the latter are patient selections based on their individual history of response or the response shown in a study lead-in period. An example is the exclusion of (likely) placebo responders. But the success of this approach seems to be variable and most likely dependent on specific features of the selection process and study design (Faries et al., 2001; Trivedi and Rush, 1995). One of these features is the duration of the run-in treatment period for evaluating placebo response; another is the type of blinding procedures used (e.g. single-blind vs double-blind run-in period; additional blinding of site investigators to the timing of response assessment and randomisation to the pivotal study phase). Promising in helping to identify more homogeneous patient groups and 'filter out' placebo responders for efficacy trials seems to be specific types of adaptive study designs such as the 'sequential parallel comparison design' (Fava et al., 2003). Similarly promising, especially for paediatric psychopharmacology trials, could be study designs in which patients receive a combination of (single-blind) placebo treatment and a psychosocial intervention in the initial study period. Only patients who fail to show a response in this period will qualify for the subsequent decisive double-blind treatment phase that compares active drug versus placebo. This approach appears to be particularly useful in those areas of child and adolescent psychiatry where treatment guidelines recommend psychotherapy as first-line treatment (for further details and a more thorough discussion, see chapter on 'Study Design' of this book). A final conclusion on the value of these relatively recent suggestions to reduce 'true' variance of therapeutic effects and exclude 'true' placebo response has to wait for more data, especially from ongoing or new paediatric psychopharmacology studies.

Finally, in order to reduce the risk of indiscriminative (false-negative) efficacy studies, major efforts are needed to minimise the error variance of efficacy assessments. Helpful measures and strategies involve repeated training of site raters that improves both interview and scoring skills, an increased standardisation of assessments by using structured (rather than unstructured or semistructured) clinical rating interviews, central monitoring of local site ratings and rater trends, and central ratings (Kobak et al., 2005). The usefulness of some of these measures is still subject to controversial discussions (see, e.g., the discussion on the usefulness of central ratings and structured interviews: Khan et al., 2014a,b, 2017; Kobak et al., 2007). More data from systematic prospective investigations are required that compare the impact of these measures with traditional rating methods. In addition, study monitoring needs to focus on protocol violations, deviations from standardisation rules, and possible rater trends (see also chapter on 'Running Clinical Trials' of this book). Publications on increased placebo response rates over decades (Bridge et al., 2009; Khan et al., 2017; Walsh et al., 2002) have pointed to the association between the risk of failed, false-negative studies, the magnitude of placebo response, and the number of study sites (as well as the number of patients per site). As discussed before, the number of sites and countries involved in a trial tends to increase the issue of error variance and to decrease the reliability of assessments. This is likely to be more pronounced the more heterogeneous the sites and countries are. In order to overcome this issue, patient sample sizes of clinical efficacy studies have been constantly increased over years to compensate for the larger outcome measure variances and to give studies an adequate statistical power. This seems to have created a vicious circle because larger sample sizes require even more study sites (and countries) to conduct and complete a trial within a reasonable time frame, and this is likely to further enhance the issue of unreliable assessments and error variance. In a review of these trends for adult trials with antidepressants, Khan and Brown (2015) come to the conclusion that an ideal study that avoids an enhanced risk of high placebo response rates and a false-negative outcome should include approximately 120 randomised depressed patients per treatment arm and involve not more than 12 investigational sites. In case of a two-arm study (active drug vs placebo), this would mean an average of 20 randomised and evaluable patients per site. The two successful fluoxetine studies in children and adolescents, described earlier, did meet (or come near to) these recommendations. Depending on the clinical indication, the patient population, the expected effect sizes, the required number of patients, and the study sites are likely to vary, but the general message of the earlier recommendations is that for successful clinical trials, the number of sites would ideally range from approximately 10 to 20. Current clinical phase III trials in psychopharmacology tend to involve approximately 40–60 sites or more, often distributed over 5–10 countries. Considering the high degree of competitiveness of the current clinical trial landscape but also keeping in mind that patient recruitment periods with durations over several years would have their own problems (an increasing fluctuation in study personnel which will also have an impact on error variance of assessments), a reasonable trade-off between an ideal number of study sites (and patients per site) and the time frame for patient recruitment is necessary (for more detailed and more realistic recommendations for site numbers, see the chapter on 'Running Clinical Trials in Paediatric Psychopharmacology').

The earlier recommendations for reducing the number of false-negative efficacy studies in paediatric psychopharmacology are summarised in Table 9.4.

Table 9.4 Overview of measures likely to reduce the number of indiscriminative (false-negative) efficacy studies in paediatric psychopharmacology.

Type of measure	Description of measure(s)
1. Control of patient–clinician interactions/relationship	• Investigators (especially efficacy raters) to assume neutral, research-oriented attitudes • Providing balanced study information (describing both benefits and risks) and avoiding statements likely to reinforce (unproven) health improvement expectations • Reducing the frequency and length of study assessments to a necessary minimum
2. Control of baseline score inflations	• Blinding raters for time of baseline assessment/randomisation • Using different scales for patient eligibility (for the study) and baseline (and efficacy) assessment(s)
3. Reduction of 'true' (in-group) outcome measure variance(s)	• Using patient enrichment strategies (specifically: trying to 'filter out' patients with strong placebo effects, defining a minimum disease severity threshold) • Using new study designs promising to control for placebo response (e.g. the 'sequential parallel comparison design' or a study design combining an initial psychosocial treatment phase with a subsequent double-blind phase for patients with insufficient response to psychosocial treatment)
4. Reduction of the 'error variance' of efficacy assessments/increasing the reliability of assessments	(a) Measures to enhance the reliability of assessments: • Rater selection and certification (based on clinical experience, scale experience, and knowledge of scale methodology) • Interviewer and rater training • Using structured interviews (b) Controlling for the influence of study site numbers and site distribution on the reliability of assessments: • Reduction of the number of study sites (to a necessary minimum) and increase in the number of patients per study site

9.7 Conclusion

This chapter focused on the role of placebo effects and their contribution, together with other factors, to failed efficacy studies, in particular in paediatric psychopharmacology.

The article is reflecting the perspective of a clinical researcher who is concerned about the negative impact of increasing placebo response rates and indiscriminate (false-negative) efficacy studies on drug development in psychopharmacology in general and paediatric psychopharmacology in particular. In this view, placebo effects are mainly bothersome methodological artefacts that need to be reduced or ideally even be removed. The article tried to demonstrate how a better understanding of placebo effects could help to reduce the number of failed studies.

However, an improved understanding of the sources of 'true' placebo response will not only be beneficial for drug development and research. It may also enable medical practitioners to better use the power of placebo effects for the augmentation of psychotropic drug treatment. Finally, it may also help to promote the discovery of additional and more targeted psychotherapeutic techniques and conditions. All of these expected benefits are likely to improve the chances of more effective treatment options and combinations of treatment methods for mental disorders, especially in children and adolescents.

References

Alphs, L., Benedetti, F., Fleischhacker, W.W., Kane, J.M., 2012. Placebo-related effects in clinical trials in schizophrenia: what is driving this phenomenon and what can be done to minimize it? Int. J. Neuropsychopharmacol. 15, 1003–1014. https://doi.org/10.1017/S1461145711001738.

Atkinson, S.D., Prakash, A., Zhang, Q., Pangallo, B.A., Bangs, M.E., Emslie, G.J., March, J.S., 2014. A double-blind efficacy and safety study of duloxetine flexible dosing in children and adolescents with major depressive disorder. J. Child Adolesc. Psychopharmacol. 24 (4), 180–189.

Bandura, A., 1971. Psychological Modeling: Conflicting theories. Aldine & Atherton, Chicago, IL.

Bandura, A., 1997. Self-Efficacy. The Exercise of Control. W.H. Freeman and Company, New York.

Beck, A.T., Rush, A.J., Shaw, B.F., Emery, G., 1979. Cognitive Therapy of Depression. The Guilford Press, New York.

Benedetti, F., 2014. Placebo Effects, second ed. Oxford University Press, Oxford.

Benedetti, F., Mayberg, H.S., Wagner, T.D., Stohler, C.S., Zubieta, J.-K., 2005. Neurobiological mechanisms of the placebo effect. J. Neurosci. 25 (45), 10390–10402. https://doi.org/10.1523/JNEUROSCI.3458-05.2005.

Bland, J.M., Altman, D.G., 1994. Statistics notes: regression towards the mean. Br. Med. J. 308, 1499. http://bmj.bmjjournals.com/cgi/content/full/308/6942/1499.

Bridge, J.A., Birmaher, B., Iyengar, S., Barbe, R.P., Brent, D.A., 2009. Placebo response in randomized controlled trials of antidepressants for pediatric major depressive disorder. Am. J. Psychiatry 166, 42–49.

Byrom, B., Mundt, J., 2005. The value of computer-administered self-report data in central nervous system clinical trials. Curr. Opin. Drug Discov. Devel. 8 (3), 374–383.

Choi, C.K., Pak, A.W.P., 2007. Hallo-goodbye effect. In: Salkind (Eds.), Encyclopedia of Measurement and Statistics. https://doi.org/10.4135/9781412952644.n200.

Cohen, D., Deniau, E., Maturana, A., Tanguy, M.L., Bodeau, N., Labelle, R., Brenton, J.J., Guile, J.M., 2008. Are child and adolescent responses to placebo higher in major depression than in anxiety disorders? A systematic review of placebo-controlled trials. PLoS One 3, e2632.

Cronbach, L.J., 1970. Essentials of Psychological Testing, third ed. Harper & Row, New York, Evenston, London.

De Pascalis, V., Chiaradia, C., Carotenuto, E., 2002. The contribution of suggestibility and expectation to placebo analgesia phenomenon in an experimental setting. Pain 96, 393–402.

Emslie, G.J., 2009. Understanding placebo response in pediatric depression trials. Am. J. Psychiatry 166 (1), 1–3.

Emslie, G.J., Rush, A.J., Weinberg, W.A., Kowatch, R.A., Hughes, C.W., Carmody, T., Rintelmann, J., 1997. A double-blind, randomized, placebo-controlled trial of fluoxetine in children and adolescents with depression. Arch. Gen. Psychiatry 54 (11), 1031–1037.

Emslie, G.J., Heiligenstein, J.H., Wagner, K.D., Hoog, S.L., Ernest, D.E., Brown, E., Nilsson, M., Jacobson, J.G., 2002. Fluoxetine for acute treatment of depression in children and adolescents: a placebo-controlled, randomized clinical trial. J. Am. Acad. Child Adolesc. Psychiatry 41 (10), 1205–1215.

Emslie, G.J., Ventura, D., Korotzer, A., Tourkodimitris, S., 2009. Escitalopram in the treatment of adolescent depression. A randomized placebo-controlled multisite trial. J. Am. Acad Child Adolesc. Psychiatry 48 (7), 721–729.

Emslie, G.J., Prakash, A., Zhang, Q., Pangallo, B.A., Bangs, M.A., March, J.S., 2014. A double-blind efficacy and safety study of duloxetine fixed doses in children and adolescents with major depression. J. Child Adolesc. Psychopharmacol. 24 (4), 170–179.

Ernst, E., Resch, K.L., 1995. Concept of true and perceived placebo effects. BMJ 311, 551–553.

Eysenck, M.W., Keane, M.T., 2010. Cognitive Psychology, sixth ed. Psychological Press, Hove and New York.

Faries, D.E., Heiligenstein, J.H., Tolleffson, J.H., Potter, W.Z., 2001. The double-blind variable placebo lead-in period: results from two antidepressant clinical trials. J. Clin. Psychopharmacol. 21 (6), 561–568.

Fava, M., Evins, A., Dorer, D., Schoenfeld, D., 2003. The problem of the placebo response in clinical trials for psychiatric disorders: culprits, possible remedies, and a novel study design approach. Psychother. Psychosom. 72, 115–127.

Festinger, L., 1957. A Theory of Cognitive Dissonance. Stanford Univ. Press, Stanford, CA.

Fineberg, N.A., Hawley, C.J., Gale, T.M., 2006. Are placebo-controlled trials still important for obsessive compulsive disorders? Prog. Neuro-Psychopharmacol. Biol. Psychiatry 30, 413–422.

Finniss, D.G., Kaptchuk, T.J., Miller, F., Benedetti, F., 2010. Biological, clinical, and ethical advances of placebo effects. Lancet 375, 686–695.

Fischer, G., 1974. Einführung in die Theorie Psychologischer Tests. Verlag Hans Huber, Bern, Stuttgart, Wien.

Food and Drug Administration (FDA), 2012. Guidance for Industry. Enrichment Strategies for Clinical Trials to Support Approval of Human Drugs and Biological Products. http://www.fda.gov/Drugs/GuidanceComplianceRegulatoryInformation/Guidancews/default.htm.

Geers, A.L., Miller, F.G., 2014. Understanding and translating the knowledge about placebo effects: the contribution of psychology. Curr. Opin. Psychiatry 27 (5), 326–331.

Geers, A.L., Wellman, J.A., Fowler, S.L., Helfer, S.L., France, C.R., 2010. Dispositional optimism predicts placebo analgesia. J. Pain 22, 1165–1171.

Gulliksen, H., 1950. Theory of Mental Tests. Wiley, New York.

Guy, W. (Ed.), 1976. ECDEU Assessment for Psychopharmacology. Revised Edition. National Institute of Mental Health, Rockville, MD.

Haas, M., Unis, A.S., Armenteros, J., Copenhaver, M.D., Quiroz, J.A., Kushner, S.F., 2009. A 6-week, randomized, double-blind, placebo-controlled study of the efficacy and safety of risperidone in adolescents with schizophrenia. J. Child Adolesc. Psychopharmacol. 19, 611–621.

Hazell, P., O'Connell, D., Heathcote, D., Robertson, J., Henry, D., 1995. Efficacy of tricyclic drugs in treating child and adolescent depression: a meta-analysis. BMJ 310, 897–901. https://doi.org/10.1136/bmj.310.6984.897.

Holodynski, M., Oerter, R., 2008. Tätigkeitsregulation und die entwicklung von motivation, emotion, volution. In: Oerter, R., Montada, L. (Eds.), Entwicklungspsychologie, sixth Aufl. Beltz Verlag, Weinheim, Basel, pp. 535–571.

Khan, A., Brown, W., 2015. Antidepressant versus placebo in major depression: an overview. World Psychiatry 14, 294–300.

Khan, A., Leventhal, R.M., Khan, S.R., Brown, W.A., 2002. Severity of depression and response to antidepressants and placebo: an analysis of the Food and Drug Administration database. J. Clin. Psychopharmacol. 22, 40–45.

Khan, A., Kolts, R.L., Rapaport, M.H., Krishnan, K.R., Brodhead, A.E., Browns, W.A., 2005. Magnitude of placebo response and drug-placebo differences across psychiatric disorders. Psychol. Med. 35 (5), 743–749.

Khan, A., Faucett, J., Brown, W.A., 2014a. Magnitude of placebo response and response variance in antidepressant trials using structured, taped and appraised rater interviews compared to traditional rating interviews. J. Psychiatr. Res. 51, 88–92.

Khan, A., Faucett, J., Brown, W.A., 2014b. Magnitude of change with antidepressants and placebo in antidepressant trials using structured, taped and appraised rater interview (SIGMA-RAPS) compared to trials using traditional semi-structured interviews. Psychopharmacology 231, 4301–4307.

Khan, A., Mar, K.F., Faucett, J., Khan Shilling, S., Brown, W.A., 2017. Has the rising placebo response impacted antidepressant clinical trial outcome? Data from the US Food and Drug Administration 1987-2013. World Psychiatry 16 (2), 181–192.

Kinon, B.J., Potts, A.J., Watson, S.B., 2011. Placebo response in clinical trials with schizophrenia patients. Curr. Opin. Psychiatry 24 (2), 107–113.

Kirsch, L., 1997. Specifying nonspecific: Psychological mechanisms of placebo effects. In: Harrington, A. (Ed.), The placebo effect: An interdisciplinary explanation. Harvard University Press, Cambridge, MA, pp. 166–186.

Kirsch, I., 2008. Challenging received wisdom: antidepressants and the placebo effect. McGill J. Med. 11 (2), 219–222.

Kobak, K.A., Feiger, A.D., Lipsitz, J.D., 2005. Interview quality and signal detection in clinical trials. Am. J. Psychiatry 162, 628.

Kobak, K.A., Kane, J.M., Thase, M.E., Nierenberg, A.A., 2007. Why do clinical trials fail? The problem of measurement error in clinical trials: time to test new paradigms? J. Clin. Psychopharmacol. 27, 1–5.

Landin, R., DeBrota, D.J., DeVries, T.A., Potter, W.Z., Demitrack, M.A., 2000. The impact of restrictive entry criterion during the placebo lead-in period. Biometrics 56 (1), 271–278.

Laughren, T.P., 2001. The scientific and ethical basis for placebo-controlled trials in depression and schizophrenia: an FDA perspective. Eur. Psychiatry 16, 418–423.

Leber, P., 1991. Is there an alternative to the randomized controlled trial? Psychopharmacol. Bull. 27 (1), 3–8.

Mayberg, H.S., Siolva, J.A., Brannan, S.K., Tekell, J.L., McGinnis, S., Mahurin, R.K., Jerabek, P.A., 2002. The functional neuroanatomy of the placebo effect. Am. J. Psychiatry 159, 728–737.
Montgomery, S.A., 1999. Alternatives to placebo-controlled trials in psychiatry. ECNP Consensus Meeting, Sept. 26, 1996, Amsterdam. Eur. Neuropsychopharmacol. 9, 265–269.
Montgomery, S.A., Asberg, M., 1979. A new depression scale designed to be sensitive to change. Br. J. Psychiatry 134, 382–389.
Montgomery, G., Kirsch, I., 1997. Classical conditioning and the placebo effect. Pain 72, 107–113.
Orlinsky, D.E., Howard, K.I., 1987. A generic model of psychotherapy. J. Integr. Eclectic Psychother. 6, 6–27.
Orlinsky, D.E., Ronnestad, M.E., Willutzski, U., 2004. Fifty years of psychotherapy process-outcome research: continuity and change. In: Lambert, M.J. (Ed.), Bergin and Garfield's Handbook of Psychotherapy and Behavior Change, fifth ed. John Wiley & Sons, New York.
Page, R.A., Green, J.P., 2007. An update on age, hypnotic suggestibility, and gender. A brief report. Am. J. Clin. Hypn. 49, 283–287.
Parellada, M., Moreno, C., Moreno, M., Espliego, A., De Portugal, E., Arango, C., 2012. Placebo effect in child and adolescent psychiatric trials. Eur. Neuropsychopharmacol. 22, 787–799.
Pecina, M., Bohnert, A.S., Sikora, M., Avery, E.T., Langenecker, S.A., Mickey, B.J., Zubieta, J.K., 2015. Association between placebo-activated neural systems and antidepressant responses: neurochemistry of placebo effects in major depression. JAMA Psychiatr. 72 (11), 1087–1094.
Persico, A.M., Arango, C., Buitelaar, J.K., Correll, C.U., Glennon, J.C., Hoekstra, P.J., Moreno, C., Vitiello, B., Vorstman, J., Zuddas, A., the European Child and Adolescent Clinical Psychopharmacology Network, 2015. Unmet needs in paediatric psychopharmacology: present scenario and future perspectives. Eur. Neuropsychopharmacol. 25 (10), 1513–1531.
Posternak, M.A., Zimmerman, M., 2007. Therapeutic effect of follow-up assessments on antidepressant and placebo response rates in antidepressant efficacy trials. Meta-analysis. Br. J. Psychiatry 190, 287–292.
Poznanski, E.O., Mokros, H., 1996. Children's Depression Rating Scale Revised (CDRS-R). Western Psychological Services, Los Angeles.
Poznanski, E.O., Cook, S.C., Carroll, B.J., 1979. A depression rating scale for children. Pediatrics 164, 442–450.
Prakash, A., Lobo, E., Kratochvil, C.J., Tamura, R.N., Pangallo, B.A., Bullok, K.E., Quinlan, T., Emslie, G.J., March, J.S., 2012. An open-label safety and pharmacokinetics study of duloxetine in pediatric patients with major depression. J. Child Adolesc. Psychopharmacol. 22, 48–55.
Rachman, S., 1977. The conditioning theory of fear-acquisition: a critical examination. Behav. Res. Ther. 15, 375–387.
Reynaert, C., Janne, P., Vause, M., Zhdanowicz, N., Lejeune, D., 1995. Clinical trials of antidepressants: the hidden face: where locus of control appears to play a key role in depression outcome. Psychopharmacology 119, 449–454.
Robinson, D.S., Rickels, K., 2000. Concern about clinical trials. J. Clin. Psychopharmacol. 20, 593–596.
Rogers, C.R., 1957. The necessary and sufficient conditions of therapeutic personality change. J. Consult. Psychol. 22, 95–103.
Rutherford, B.R., Roose, S.P., 2013. A model of placebo response in antidepressant clinical trials. Am. J. Psychiatry 170 (7), 723–733. https://doi.org/10.1176/appi.ajp.2012.12040474.

Rutherford, B.R., Sneed, J.R., Roose, S.P., 2009. Does study design influence outcome. The effects of placebo control and treatment duration on antidepressant trials. Psychother. Psychosom. 78, 172–181.

Rutherford, B.R., Sneed, J.R., Tandler, J., Petersen, B.S., Roose, S.P., 2011. Deconstructing pediatric depression trials: a pilot study. In: Poster Presented at the Annual Meeting of the American Psychiatric Association.

Sandler, A.D., Glesne, C., Geller, G., 2008. Children's and parents'perspectives on open-label use of placebos in the treatment of ADHD. Child Care Health Dev. 34, 111–120.

Seiffge-Krenke, I., 2008. Gesundheit als aktiver Gestaltungsprozess im menschlichen Lebenslauf. In: Oerter, T., Montada, L. (Eds.), Entwicklungspsychologie, sixth Aufl. Beltz Verlag, Weinheim, Basel, pp. 822–836.

Simmons, K., Ortiz, R., Kossowsky, J., Krummenacher, P., Grillon, C., Pine, D., Colloca, L., 2014. Pain and placebo in pediatrics: a comprehensive review of laboratory and clinical findings. Pain 155 (11), 2229–2235. https://doi.org/10.1016/j.pain.2014.08.035.

Stein, D.J., Baldwin, D.S., Dolberg, O.T., Despiegel, N., Bandelow, B., 2006. Which factors predict placebo response in anxiety disorders and major depression? An analysis of placebo-controlled studies of escitalopram. J. Clin. Psychiatry 67, 1741–1746.

Stewart-Williams, S., Podd, J., 2004. The placebo effect: dissolving the expectancy versus conditioning debate. Psychol. Bull. 130 (2), 324–340.

Tates, K., Meeuwesen, L., 2001. Doctor-parent-child communication. A (re)view of the literature. Soc. Sci. Med. 52, 839–851.

Trivedi, M., Rush, J., 1995. Does a placebo run-in or a placebo treatment cell affect the efficacy of antidepressant medications? Neuropsychopharmacology 11, 33–43.

Vervoort, T., Huguet, A., Verhoeven, K., Goubert, L., 2011. Mothers' and fathers' responses to their child's pain moderate the relationship between the child's pain catastrophizing and disability. Pain 152 (4), 786–793.

Wagner, K.D., Jonas, J., Findling, R.L., Ventura, D., Saikali, K., 2006. A double-blind, randomized, placebo-controlled trial with escitalopram in the treatment of pediatric depression. J. Am. Acad. Child Adolesc. Psychiatry 45, 280–288.

Walsh, B.T., Seidman, S.N., Sysko, R., Gould, M., 2002. Placebo response in studies with major depression: variable, substantial, and growing. JAMA 287 (14), 1840–1847.

Weimer, K., Gulewitsch, M.D., Schlarb, A.A., Schwille-Kiuntke, J., Klosterhalfen, S., Enck, P., 2013. Placebo effects in children: a review. Pediatr. Res. 74 (1), 96–102.

Wilens, T.E., Spencer, T.J., Biederman, J., 2002. A review of pharmacotherapy of adults with attention-deficit/hyperactivity disorder. J. Atten. Disord. 6, 189–202.

Yao, L., 2013. FDA Takes Step to Encourage Pediatric Drug Studies. Posted on Aug. 26, 2013 by FDA Voice, https://blogs.fda.gov/fdavoice/index.php/2013/08/fda-takes-step-to-encourage-pediatric-drug-studies/.

Further reading

Mayberg, H.S., 2003. Modulating dysfunctional limbic-cortical circuits in depression: towards development of brain-based algorithms for diagnosis and optimized treatment. Br. Med. Bull. 65, 193–207.

Running clinical trials in paediatric psychopharmacology

Klaudius Siegfried[†]
Goethe Univ. Frankfurt, Frankfurt, Germany

10.1 Introduction

The focus of this article will be on *study management tasks, operational challenges, and considerations* associated with the planning, setup, and running of paediatric psychopharmacology trials. The objectives of these tasks are to implement and run the study according to the directions and requirements of the study protocol. Therefore the prerequisite for an initiation of these tasks is the availability of at least an outline of essential features of the study protocol. Not all operational steps and tasks will be discussed but mainly those that are likely to pose *specific challenges for paediatric psychopharmacology studies*. As an introduction the first section will provide a short general overview of essential study management tasks. In subsequent sections, challenges particularly associated with the implementation and running of paediatric psychopharmacology studies will be discussed and possible solutions proposed.

10.2 Overview of essential study management tasks and the operational plan

Study management involves the planning, directing, and monitoring of all operational tasks and activities of a study project, related to its setup, implementation, conduct, and completion. 'Operational tasks' are defined by specific types of activities required to achieve the defined project goals and help to 'translate' protocol requirements into actions. When defining these actions and goals, it is also necessary to determine the project timelines and identify the resources, required to successfully conduct and complete the tasks. 'Resources' include both the number and type of people needed for the various tasks and other resources (such as specific equipment and financial resources). Careful project planning is an essential prerequisite for running projects successfully. The core of project planning is an 'operational plan' and ongoing adaptive corrections of features of this plan in view of changing or not adequately anticipated conditions. As will be shown in subsequent sections of this article, successful planning and adaptive corrections require a good understanding of the disease and patient population under investigation, the current standard of care in the countries selected for the study, and the operational implications of study protocol features. The operational plan involves a

---

[†]Deceased.

flowchart of (parallel and sequential) project tasks; the study timelines; and objectives and action plans for each tasks necessary to setup, implement, conduct, and complete the study as well as plans for data evaluation and reporting the study results. Important features of the operational plan include the following (highlighted by bullet points):

- *Study timelines* (for each study phase and the study as a whole): The overall timelines will depend on realistic expectations and commercial goals. They are usually part of a clinical development plan, a strategic plan that includes all necessary studies (phase I, II, and III) until submission of the study reports to regulatory bodies for registration or new drug application (NDA). In order for study timelines to be realistic, they need to be based on relevant information about the target patient population and the disease under investigation. This specifically includes prevalence and incidence of the disease, possible obstacles in patient recruitment that may operate as filters for the number of patients available for the planned study, and current standard treatment ('standard of care')—its benefits, adverse events, and unmet medical needs. In addition the number of suitable investigational sites has to be taken into account. The suggested timelines need to be supported by adequate feasibility assessments (see in the succeeding text).
- *A site and country distribution plan* and *a (patient) recruitment plan*:
  - *Country and site distribution plan*: This plan needs to address the following questions: Where, that is, at which type of study sites, can the defined patient group be found? Which type of investigators (specifically: which medical specialties) are needed? Which type of (other) study personnel and site equipment is needed (e.g. raters for specific clinical scales and centrifuges for certain lab values)? Do the investigators and the other site personnel have to meet additional selection criteria (e.g. years of study experience, familiarity/experience with certain types of rating scales, and familiarity with specific types of studies)? What is the percentage of newly diagnosed, untreated patients with the disease in question that visit the study centres per month (or within 6 or 12 months)? Can patients that are already under another treatment be switched to the study treatment, and under which conditions could this occur? How many of such patients would be available at the study sites? Can the study site realistically commit to recruit a minimum number of x patients within a defined timeframe (e.g. of 1 year or 2)? Are there differences in recruitment rates between possibly suitable study sites, regions, and countries? What is the expected screen failure rate, and which type of screen failures are likely to occur and drive this rate? Considering the required sample size of randomised patients, how many patients need to be screened for the study and (on average) per study site? How many study sites would be needed to recruit the necessary number of screened and randomised patients? Are there preferred countries where the study sites should be placed (e.g. in view of the registration plans for the drug, possible marketing plans, and the overall study timelines and data quality)? Can the study be conducted in one single country, or does it need to be distributed over several countries? What are the advantages and disadvantages of possible countries (e.g. in terms of study approval conditions, recruitment rates/speed of recruitment, reputation, experience of investigators/sites, and expected data quality)? What is the expected date of the 'first patient in the study' and the 'last patient out'?
  - *Specific recruitment strategy questions*: Is competitive recruitment acceptable, or a modified, more restricted competitive recruitment strategy needed? Can/should patient recruitment be supported by site support measures and specific recruitment initiatives, for example, patient advertising, and, if so, is this acceptable in the selected countries? Are specific types of advertising material needed, including translations and adaptations of this material, and are sufficient financial resources for advertising campaigns and material available?

- *Feasibility assessments and final site and country selection*: The operational plan needs to be supported by a specific feasibility study conducted in a representative sample of study sites. The feasibility study needs to obtain relevant information regarding the availability of suitable patients, the acceptability of study requirements and patients' and investigators' interest in participating in the planned study, patient recruitment and screen failure rates, and the required number of sites and countries. The feasibility assessments require interviews with sites or the completion of standardised feasibility questionnaires by the study sites (or a combination of both). The value of the feasibility findings will depend on the type of questions asked, in particular whether or not all relevant critical conditions for patient recruitment and study conduct have been adequately addressed. Examples are specific inclusion and exclusion criteria (e.g. minimum severity of disease, prohibited or allowable co-morbid conditions, specific patient history features, and inpatient/outpatient status), study design features (length of wash-out and treatment periods; acceptability of placebo controlled or other types of study plans; and add-on studies (adjunctive to a recognised treatment) vs monotherapy (placebo-controlled) studies, frequency of study visits, and number and length of assessments per visit day), and types of prohibited and allowable previous and concomitant medication and other concomitant treatment (e.g. certain types of psychotherapy). A basic prerequisite of feasibility studies is that the sample of study sites selected is representative for the available (population of) study sites. If this prerequisite is not met, the obtained feasibility findings will not have sufficient predictive validity and will therefore be inadequate for a decision on the final country and site distribution. Since there will be variations between sites in terms of recruitment rates, experience, and other features and these variations need to be represented in the feasibility study site sample, it is necessary that feasibility studies comprise a significantly larger number of potential study sites and countries than the finally required number. This will also allow for the final country and site distribution the selection of a subset of sites and countries that are likely to be most suitable in terms of the overall study objectives. The final country and site distribution plan, based on the obtained feasibility information, need to be compared with the initially expected patient recruitment and overall study timeline plans in order to find out whether the initial timelines can be met or need some modification. In case of major discrepancies between expected and obtained recruitment rates, it may become necessary to modify study timelines and/or to reconsider critical features of the study protocol. In the latter case, it needs to be discussed whether the required protocol modifications will be scientifically and methodologically acceptable or could compromise the study quality.
- *Planning of regulatory and Institutional Review Board (IRB)/Ethics Committee (EC) submissions and study approvals*: Important questions to be addressed in this context are the following: Which countries are to be considered for the study? Which are the typical submission and approval timelines in these countries? Are there critical submission dates (e.g. at the end of each month)? How many days, weeks, or months are typically needed to receive approval by regulatory authorities in the countries considered? Are these timelines likely to vary with the type of study (e.g. study population and study design)? Do authorities in certain countries have specific requirements and concerns or a specific focus in their reviews of study documents (e.g. concerns about placebo-controlled studies and specific concerns and requirements regarding studies in children)? What types of documents are needed for a submission? Is the translation of specific documents required? Several of the earlier questions also apply to EC/IRB submissions (e.g. submission timelines, focus of review, concerns, documents required). In addition, one needs to consider the advantages and disadvantages of using centralised IRBs/ECs, and which centralised IRB/EC would be best to select. It is useful to anticipate questions and concerns of regulatory authorities and IRBs/ECs and

proactively consider possible measures to address these questions and concerns (e.g. by submitting additional information material, which is likely to facilitate and speed up the approval process). There are significant differences in approval timelines of various regulatory authorities and IRBs/ECs. It is therefore unrealistic to assume that all sites and countries selected for a study will be able to start with the study at the same time. Therefore differences in the length of approval timelines need to be incorporated in the patient recruitment plan.

Monitoring study progress and ongoing projections for the completion of study tasks: The operational plan outlined earlier is a living document throughout the course of a project. For each of the study tasks—the modules of the project plan—the actual start, progress, and completion times have to be carefully monitored and compared with the planned times. Reasons for discrepancies between planned and actual timelines need to be evaluated and corrective actions be considered, decided, and implemented. If applicable, new, modified timelines will be needed.

A fairly complex task is the monitoring of patient recruitment activities and study conduct issues in multicentre studies. Specific electronic systems that can store, summarise, and evaluate relevant data on various levels—individual study site, country, and study level—are very valuable tools in monitoring changes, issues and hurdles, and progress. They allow quick and effective corrective actions. Traditional individual site monitoring is still important but needs to be supplemented and supported by central monitoring (based on electronic case record form (CRF) data).

The preceding text was a general outline of essential operational tasks and study management responsibilities. All of these do, of course, also apply to studies in paediatric psychopharmacology. The following sections will be dedicated to challenges that frequently occur in paediatric psychopharmacology trials.

10.3 The impact of attitudes towards paediatric psychopharmacology trials on patient availability and recruitment

Attitudes towards medical treatment and clinical studies can foster and facilitate the conduct of clinical trials or make it more difficult, even unfeasible. Of particular relevance in this context are attitudes of the target patient groups and (in case of paediatric patients) parents (or legal representatives) and those of potential clinical investigators. These attitudes are often strongly influenced and shaped by mass media (television and radio programmes and newspapers/magazines) and social networks.

In case of paediatric psychopharmacology studies, the attitudes of the clinical trial subjects, especially when children, will be mostly dependent on what they hear and learn from their parents about clinical studies and the risks and benefits associated with the participation in such studies. Unfortunately, in some countries and regions, the attitudes of parents towards clinical studies in children and adolescents are negatively influenced by the mass media. The impression is created that subjects are used in clinical studies as 'guinea pigs' and pharmaceutical companies do not care about the well-being of patients but are mainly interested in profit making. This is likely to sensitise parents and make them critical and cautious towards the participation of their children/adolescents in such studies. This will be an even more critical issue in case of drug studies in children and adolescents with psychological disorders because, in the public opinion, psychotherapy is often believed to be more adequate and drug treatment as potentially harmful. Even parents with less negative attitudes may become hesitant to allow their children to participate in studies because they do not want to appear in the opinion of their friends and neighbours as bad parents who do not sufficiently care about the safety and well-being of their children. The frequency and strength of negative attitudes towards clinical studies varies across countries and appears to be also dependent on the type of the local health-care system: subjects in countries in which everybody has a health insurance use to have much different attitudes towards clinical studies than those from countries in which a major part of the population has no health insurance or where the available insurance allows only access to a selected group of cheaper, which often means: older medication. For subjects/parents from the latter two types of countries, participation in clinical studies is usually more valuable in that it gives them access to treatment they otherwise may never be able to receive or afford. In contrast, in countries, where everybody has a health insurance, there are much less incentives for participating in drug studies, especially in placebo-controlled studies (which involve the risk of not receiving active drug treatment).

Favourable attitudes towards clinical psychopharmacology studies in children and adolescents are likely to be found in representatives of major regulatory agencies (such as the US Food and Drug Administration (FDA) in the United States and the European Medicines Agency (EMA) in Europe), leading experts in child and adolescent psychiatry and in a majority of paediatric psychiatrists. These groups emphasise the need of having more systematic research projects in paediatric psychopharmacology. There is, however, a subgroup of paediatric specialists that have some reservations towards drug treatment for mental disorders in children and (though to a lesser extent) adolescents. These are usually physicians and psychologists with a background in psychotherapy and psychological theories of paediatric psychopathology, particularly psychodynamically trained paediatric specialists.

The described negative attitudes and reservations against drug studies in children and adolescents, especially with psychiatric disorders, are an important factor that accounts for the number of interested investigators and study sites as well as the number of parents who are willing to let their children participate in such studies. Experience has shown that favourably motivated but unexperienced clinical investigators often underestimate the difficulties finding larger numbers of patients for their study because they underestimate the impact of unfavourable attitudes towards drug studies.

The earlier description of the 'environment' for paediatric psychopharmacology studies is not meant to discourage sponsors and clinicians from planning studies in paediatric psychopharmacology but to increase awareness of these difficulties and consider appropriate measures to improve this situation. More than in other areas of clinical drug studies, it appears to be important in paediatric psychopharmacology to better inform the public by providing more relevant information and training about treatment options and the value of clinical trials. When planning such studies, it is recommended to select early on, in each of the countries considered for the trial(s), leading medical specialists to discuss what could be done to make studies more acceptable and which way would be the possibly most effective. These experts could also function as opinion leaders in their country, to speak up in the public (e.g. in interviews in radio or television programmes); publish in local newspaper; and give lectures to their medical colleagues and their staff about the disease in question, the treatment options, and the need and usefulness of good efficacy and safety studies. The primary purpose of such activities would be to help creating a medically better informed public, which is an important basis for more favourable attitudes towards clinical trials in paediatric psychopharmacology. It is important to involve local experts from ideally all countries supposed to participate in a study and not only a small group of international experts. Local experts know what approach (presentations and involvement of newspapers, TV, and other) will work best in their country and region. In addition, they speak the local language, which is a prerequisite for talking to target patient groups or their parents. The involvement of leading local medical specialists (as investigators or members of a study advisory committee) is likely to enhance the credibility and acceptability of the study project, to facilitate local regulatory and IRB/EC approval, and to convince hesitant clinicians to participate in the planned study as investigators.

10.4 Challenges in the approval of studies by local regulatory authorities and IRBs/ECs

The investigation of new psychotropic drugs in paediatric populations is strongly recommended and promoted by major regulatory authorities, in particular by the FDA and the EMA. However, this strong support is not always shared by local regulatory bodies and IRBs/ECs. Possible reservations and critical attitudes are usually driven by a mixture of concerns, associated with good intentions about a special protection of 'fragile subjects' (like children), and a lack of knowledge about the value of specific types of studies in the target population. The latter is likely to occur if the IRB/EC members are not familiar with paediatric indications, especially in paediatric psychopharmacology. Reservations come most frequently up in discussions of placebo-controlled drug studies in children and adolescents. Unfortunately, placebo-controlled studies are indispensable as key evidence for efficacy of drugs in psychopharmacology (see chapter on Indiscriminative Efficacy Trials and Placebo Effects). In discussions with local authorities or IRBs/ECs, it is usually not sufficient to simply refer to FDA or EMA guidance documents. The most effective way to convince them is to create concise informational material, a list of arguments supporting the approval of such studies. These need to include the following:

(a) A reference to the relevant FDA and EMA clinical guidelines for drug development in this specific clinical indication. In addition, if applicable, a statement (with supportive documents) that the study protocol was discussed and agreed with the FDA and/or EMA.
(b) A paper that briefly summarises the usefulness and necessity of placebo-controlled studies for a convincing proof of efficacy, in particular, in areas like paediatric psychopharmacology

that are characterised by substantial placebo effects, which vary with therapeutic settings and studies. An explicit quote of the high placebo responder rates in paediatric psychopharmacology studies appears to be useful in this context (see chapter on 'Indiscriminative Efficacy Studies and Placebo Effects...' in this book). Such figures may not only be helpful in illustrating the extent of placebo effects but also soften concerns about the lack of possible benefits of the placebo group.

(c) A list of measures for protecting patients' safety in the planned study. The list needs to include specific study regulations such as precise instructions for parents/patients when to contact the study site in case of potentially critical events, frequent patient contacts by site personnel (e.g. regular telephone calls in-between study visits focusing on potential safety issues), clear rules on study discontinuation, and rescue medication in case of safety concerns. Finally, it is worthwhile pointing out in a specific note that, as a rule, in clinical trials subjects are more thoroughly examined and medically supervised (in terms of thoroughness, frequency, and length of medical assessments and visits) than patients in everyday clinical practice.

Sometimes, local authorities and IRBs/ECs, depending on the expertise of their staff, may also raise questions about available preclinical data and pharmacological and toxicological findings that support the use and safety of the test drug in children and adolescents. This includes questions on potential drug effects on developmental processes, modifications of metabolism, and pharmacokinetic parameters in paediatric populations (as compared with adults). In case of submissions for phase III trials, questions could be specifically asked about pharmacokinetic and safety data from a phase II clinical study in children/adolescents and the basis of the dose selection for the planned paediatric trial.

A major focus of IRBs/ECs will be on the contents and wording of the parents' informed consent and the children's assent forms. Both need to be obtained for paediatric studies, though country and state laws differ in their definition on who constitutes a 'child' and from which year of age onwards a person can legally consent to participate in a study. The 'informed consent', to be provided by parents, is an agreement by someone who has the legal capacity to give consent and who exercises free power of choice to participate in a study. In order to make an informed decision, the person must have sufficient knowledge and understanding of the research in question as well as of the anticipated risks and benefits (Levine, 1988). (Informed) 'Assent' is a child's agreement and express of willingness to participate and cooperate in a study. It is to be obtained (in addition to parents' informed consent) by subjects that are by definition (of the respective state/country) too young to give informed consent (Levy et al., 2003). Information provided for the child's assent is supposed to help him/her to understand that he/she is asked to participate in a (research) study, that he/she can speak to anybody about this study and his/her participation in it before giving his/her assent, and, finally, that he/she can withdraw from the study at any time without disadvantages. The purpose of the study needs to be explained and its (diagnostic, efficacy, and safety) procedures to be described as well as its possible benefits and risks. Important in the IRB's/EC's review of the assent text will be the appropriateness of the language and wording to the child's age and development level. The explanations of procedures and medical concepts are to be given in simple language. Medical terminology is to be avoided. The child/adolescent should easily understand what is expected from him/her. In order to avoid questions and queries on appropriate language and wording of assent texts, it is advisable to ask clinicians who are experienced with children of the specific age groups to review and modify the texts. For texts used in international, multicountry/multilanguage studies, it is recommendable to let the translations (of the usual English master versions) into local languages review by native speakers that are experienced with children. Literal translations of the original language texts are sometimes inadequate and need to be adapted in the translation. In case of smaller children, it often facilitates their understanding when some informative pictures are added, which illustrate the study procedures.

IRBs/ECs often also review the clinical scales foreseen for the planned study. Again the focus will be on the type of questions asked and the appropriateness of the language in which they are asked. Local translations of these scales will therefore be required for submission and may become subject of discussions. When there are published validated standard versions of the original scale and validated local language translations/adaptations, most queries can be sufficiently addressed by pointing out that these questions and scales have been empirically tested and validated for their appropriateness in the age group(s) in question.

A major hurdle for the approval of a paediatric psychopharmacology study by local authorities and IRBs/ECs can be discrepancies between local treatment guidelines and study requirements. Most frequently, this occurs in those areas of paediatric psychopharmacology where the local treatment guidelines recommend psychotherapy as first-line treatment, whereas the study protocol does not foresee psychotherapy and may even explicitly exclude psychotherapeutic treatment immediately prior to study start. Possible solutions of this issue are the following: to accept previous psychotherapeutic treatment (even immediately before entering the study), provided patients have been for the last 8 or 12 weeks on a stable treatment regimen (i.e. the same amount of hours per week for psychotherapeutic sessions) and have shown an insufficient response to this treatment. One may even consider allowing the continuation of previous psychotherapeutic treatment throughout the study, provided there is no change in its intensity and frequency and an insufficient clinical response has been shown. Another solution could be to formally foresee an initial study phase with a defined, standardised brief psychosocial treatment, which every patient has to undergo.

10.5 Considerations on patient recruitment times and country and site selection

Over the last decades, patient sample sizes of clinical psychopharmacology studies have been steadily increased. This trend was described for antidepressant trials in adults (Khan et al., 2017; Walsh et al., 2002) and also for paediatric depression studies (Bridge et al., 2009) but represents a fairly generalised tendency applicable to almost all areas of psychopharmacology. In paediatric depression trials, published between January 1988 and July 2006, the sample sizes per treatment arm ranged from approximately 50 to 180 randomised patients, with increasing numbers in more recent studies. There were significant correlations between the year of publication of these studies, their placebo response rates, risk of study failure, and the increasing number of study sites per study (Bridge et al., 2009). (For more detailed information, see chapter on 'The Issue of Indiscriminative Efficacy Trials and Placebo Effects in Paediatric Psychopharmacology'.) The ever increasing patient sample sizes are attempts to secure the chance of reaching the level of statistical significance for an observed treatment effect. But, unfortunately, these attempts have created an increasing dilemma that could be described as a vicious circle, which does not solve the issue but is likely to make it worse over time:

- Increases in study sample sizes inevitably require longer patient recruitment times or larger numbers of study sites (or both). Furthermore the ever increasing numbers of studies in recent years have created a competitive landscape that makes it even more difficult to conduct studies within a reasonable timeframe and to find a sufficient number of suitable study sites. Recruitment periods for large phase III studies in paediatric psychopharmacology studies currently comprise about 12–24 months. These recruitment periods result in overall study periods of approximately 3–3½ years.
- Faced with the issue of increasing patient sample sizes, sponsors are hesitant to prolong overall study times beyond 3–4 years and prefer an increase in the number of participating study sites. Increases in the number of study sites bring about further increases in competition with other concurrently running studies. Typical consequences of this competition are the decreases in the (average) number of recruited and randomised patients per study site, inclusion of more countries, and less experienced investigators and sites. Unfortunately, all of these measures are likely to have a negative impact on the interrater reliability of assessments and error variance component of outcome measures and thus make it more difficult to obtain statistically significant treatment effects.
- In order to prevent statistically insignificant treatment differences, sample sizes are often further increased for the next studies.

So obviously, increases in patient samples lead to the inclusion of more study sites and countries and these, in turn, to smaller average patient samples per study site, increased placebo response, and all of this results in an enhanced risk of indiscriminative false-negative studies (i.e. studies that fail to demonstrate efficacy for efficacious drugs). The described situation is typical for all clinical psychopharmacology studies because of their usually high placebo responder rates and the nature of outcome measures used. For paediatric trials, this issue is even more pronounced for the following reasons: First, with some exceptions (e.g. attention deficit hyperactivity disorder (ADHD)), prevalence rates of mental disorders in children and adolescents are lower than in adults, which means that less patients are available for clinical drug studies and recruitment rates tend to be lower than in adult studies. Second, given the relatively short history of large clinical development programmes and studies in paediatric psychopharmacology (in comparison with drug development in adult populations), the number of experienced clinical investigators ('first-tier investigators') is more limited for paediatric psychopharmacology studies than for studies in adults. As a consequence, it is often inevitable to include larger subgroups of relatively inexperienced investigators and sites. The involvement of inexperienced investigators, however, increases the risk of less reliable ratings. There are two complementary types of measures to reduce the described risk of study failure:

(a) The first is related to considerations on the *desirable number of study sites*.
(b) The second to the *selection process for less experienced investigators*.

Considerations and recommendations on the desirable number of study sites: In consideration of the described trends and risks of placebo response rates and failed studies with antidepressants and after carefully reviewing the factors accounting for these trends, clinical researchers (Khan and Brown, 2015; Rutherford and Roose, 2013) offered the following recommendations to enhance the success for pivotal studies in (adult) depression:

(1) Patients sample sizes of approximately 120 patients per treatment arm are required.
(2) The number of study sites needs to be restricted to 10–12 sites per study.

The latter is applicable to studies with two treatment arms, active drug and placebo. Ten to twelve study sites would in this case mean an average number of 20–24 randomised patients per study site. This is quite a demanding requirement, in particular when considering that there will be a screen failure rate. In order to have 20–24 randomised patients, a study site would need to screen approximately 30–34 potentially suitable patients. Obviously, these numbers will vary with the type of the investigated disorders, but, tentatively, a range of 10–20 sites per study would be the ideal number of sites for most clinical indications in psychopharmacology. These recommendations would be even more challenging for paediatric psychopharmacology studies, given the usually lower prevalence rates of many paediatric mental disorders and the relatively low number of experienced study sites. The specific challenge for paediatric psychopharmacology studies is that, on one hand, due to the higher placebo responder rates in paediatric populations, a restriction in the number of study sites appears to be even more important for paediatric psychopharmacology than for adult trials. However, on the other hand, a rigorous restriction of the number of sites could endanger the feasibility of paediatric studies. Therefore more realistic recommendations are needed that represent a good compromise based on a pragmatic trade-off between methodological requirements, on one hand, and the feasibility considerations, on the other. It is difficult to suggest modified realistic recommendations without sufficient empirical evidence that can support them. Such data are, unfortunately, not available. Therefore the following modified recommendations, which are based on trade-off considerations described earlier, are proposed as preliminary guidelines:

- For most clinical indications (e.g. studies of patients with depressive disorders, anxiety disorders, schizophrenia, and ADHD), the patient sample sizes for pivotal studies need to be in the range of approximately 100–120 (randomised) patients per treatment arm. Studies with more than three treatment arms should be avoided because their total sample sizes would need a considerably much larger number of study sites.
- Each study site should have at least three, ideally four patients per study arm. This would mean a minimum total number of 6 to, ideally, 8 randomised patients per site in case of a 2-arm study or 9 to, ideally, 12 in case of 3-arm studies. These numbers do not include the number of screen failures, which, depending on the clinical indication, are likely to be in a range of approximately 20%–40%!

- The preceding text would require a total of approximately 30 sites per study. This number could be reduced when allowing for recruitment periods of approximately 2–3 years.
- The number of the involved countries needs to be kept as low as possible, not larger than three to five. The selection of countries with similar cultures and languages is preferable. Larger language and cultural differences are associated with larger differences in word connotations of scale instructions and scale items and in the appropriateness and social desirability of behaviour assessed in scale items. These differences are likely to have an impact on the efficacy ratings. They affect the comparability/equivalence of language versions of clinical scales in culturally different countries. As a result the overall interrater reliability of assessments for a study that tends to decrease the more heterogeneous countries will be involved. Each country needs to be represented by at least three study sites, better five. This is not only for logistical and financial reasons—obviously more countries mean also more regulatory submissions, translations of documents, negotiations with different regulatory bodies, and different study timelines. There are also good methodological reasons for having more than two sites per country. In case of differences between a single site or two sites in a specific country and the rest of the study sites, it cannot be determined whether these differences reflect random or rather systematic variations. (Note: The earlier rule on country selection does not prohibit the use of a different group of (culturally similar) countries for a second study that might be needed for cross validation.)

Strategy for selecting additional less experienced investigators/sites: If 30 sites (or more) will be needed for a paediatric psychopharmacology study, the number of available highly experienced sites/investigators and networks will most likely not be sufficient. Therefore the following strategy is recommended for the selection of additional study sites and investigators:

(a) Select as many investigators/sites as possible that are experienced in conducting studies in the paediatric target population.
(b) The (additional) selection of less experienced investigators should be performed in collaboration with the already selected experienced investigators and networks. The latter should be asked to recommend other colleagues and be available for their training and support throughout the study.

Obviously, the earlier recommendations will have an impact on feasibility studies for study planning. Even the modified recommendations are fairly challenging when considering that in most phase III pivotal paediatric psychopharmacology, 40 and more study sites are involved. But a restriction in the number of study sites with a slight extension of recruitment times to approximately 2–3 years is likely to reduce the risk of study failure.

10.6 Considerations on patient recruitment strategies

The previous section already discussed the duration of recruitment periods. This section will focus on recruitment strategies and aids.

- *Competitive* vs *noncompetitive patient recruitment*: Competitive recruitment has the advantage of allowing each study site to recruit as many patients as possible and as quickly as possible, depending on the availability of suitable patients. This is, as a rule, the fastest way to reach the overall recruitment goal. Its disadvantage is that it can result in large discrepancies in sample sizes between individual study sites—with one extreme subgroup of sites having many patients and another extreme subgroup with only a few or no patients by the time the overall recruitment goal is reached. Such discrepancies do not only cause problems for the statistical evaluation but also tend to decrease the overall reliability of outcome measures and increase their variances. This may endanger the successful demonstration of a statistically significant treatment effect. It was therefore recommended earlier that each study site needs to have a defined minimum of (randomised) patients. This restriction does not completely prohibit competitive recruitment. But, in order to allow slower recruiting sites to make their required contribution, one needs also to define a maximum patient number per site for well-recruiting sites. The latter does not require a rigid a priori definition but can be dynamically adapted to the progression of the recruitment process both on the overall study level and on the site level. In any case, such rules can lead to a temporary hold or full stop of recruitment activities for rapidly recruiting sites—and that could mean not only a deceleration of recruitment but also an extension of the recruitment period.

- *Recruitment with stratified patient subgroups*: For paediatric psychopharmacology studies that plan to include male and female children and adolescents, it is useful to stratify these subgroups by defining either a minimum proportion by which each groups needs to be represented in the study sample or even fixed proportions for each patient subgroup. (For further discussion, see section on 'Considering Operational Consequences of Study Protocol Features'.) The downside of such stratifications is that they will impose further restrictions on competitive recruitment and thereby slow down the patient recruitment process. Obviously, the more stratification dimensions are foreseen by a study protocol, the more pronounced will be the impact on the speed of recruitment. In order to minimise the (negative) impact of stratifications on the overall patient recruitment time, it is necessary to select stratification rules that are consistent with known prevalence rates of the patient subgroups and adapt the required recruitment period (and/or the number of required study sites) accordingly. For example, depression (MDD) occurs approximately in 2% of children and 4%–8% of adolescents (American Academy of Child and Adolescent Psychiatry, 1998; Emslie et al., 2002). In addition, in depressed children, the prevalence rates of male and female patients are comparable, whereas in adolescents the male–female distribution is 2:1, similar as in adults (Fegert and Kölch, 2011). It is therefore unrealistic to expect that within the same timeframe in the same number of depressed children and adolescents and among adolescents, the same proportion of male and female patients can be recruited by the same number of study sites.

- *The role of advertising in boosting patients' recruitment rates*: Advertising for clinical studies, including for paediatric psychopharmacology studies, can help in boosting recruitment rates. This could be achieved by using multiple public media and types of material. Worldwide, the role of modern social media (e.g. Facebook, WhatsApp, and Twitter) has become more and more prominent as effective advertising tools. When planning advertising campaigns, the following needs to be taken into consider. First, advertising is not allowed in all countries. Second, the advertising material needs to be approved by IRBs/ECs—which may cost extra time. Third, among those countries where advertising is allowed, both the impact and the usefulness of different communication media and types of informational material are likely to vary. In order to accomplish optimal effects, it is advisable to tailor the use of advertising techniques and material according to the needs of individual study sites and regions by discussing with them the various options and offering a set of methods and material and allowing them to make their own choices.

When utilising advertising for patient recruitment one needs, however, also to consider some caveats: first, advertising usually results in significant higher screen failure rates, which may become a real burden for study sites and therefore require additional help, for example, a telephone prescreening service. Second, the core of many advertising techniques is raising specific expectations of incentives and benefits when entering and participating in a clinical trial. The stronger these expectations, the more likely they will promote placebo effects, which need to be avoided (see chapter on 'The Issue of Indiscriminative Efficacy Trials and Placebo Effects…' in this book). Since many groups and companies specialised in recruitment techniques for clinical trials are usually also offering a package of 'patient recruitment and retention techniques' (to help keeping patients in a study and reducing early drop-out rates), it appears appropriate to add in this context a specific comment on retention techniques: These are useful measures when they focus on reminders (i.e. not to forget scheduled study visits) and facilitate patient visits (e.g. compensation of travelling costs to study sites and availability of beverages and snacks at or in the neighbourhood of study sites). However, strong motivation to visit the study site and stay in the study is certainly a source of placebo effects, and the reduction of differential drop-out rates between treatment arms (e.g. between active drug and placebo treatment) is likely to 'wipe off' relevant treatment differences and thereby increase the risk of study failure. The advice is therefore to carefully consider the pros and cons of utilised recruitment and retention techniques by giving a preference to techniques that are focusing on patient information and facilitating travelling to and staying at study sites.

In order for recruitment plans and techniques to be successful and reach the goals outlined in the recruitment plan, ongoing regular checks of recruitment rates, screen failure rates, and reasons for screen failures throughout the entire recruitment period will be essential. This will need to happen on different levels—the level of individual study sites, country, and the overall study level. Discrepancies between projected and real recruitment figures will require the analysis of root causes, attempt to modify and remove these causes, and update recruitment projections. (For further details, see the sections on 'Considering Operational Consequences of Study Protocol Features' and 'Study Monitoring' of this chapter.)

10.7 Considering operational consequences of study protocol features

'Operational consequences' of study protocol features refer to the impact of study protocol requirements on study feasibility, that is, on patient recruitment, drop-out rates, and study timelines. Protocol requirements with a significant impact on study feasibility need special attention in study planning and monitoring. Ideally, such consequences are anticipated before the study protocol is finalised and approved, and the study has started. But in case of the occurrence of unexpected significant feasibility issues and hurdles during the study, it will be necessary to discuss the pros and cons of study protocol modifications and amendments. The protocol features discussed in the following are likely to have a significant impact on the feasibility of a study, especially in paediatric psychopharmacology. In the context of this discussion, some of the topics reviewed in previous sections will need to be readdressed and further discussed under a slightly different perspective.

- *The impact of co-morbidity on patient recruitment*: Co-morbidity, that is, the co-occurrence of two or more conditions, defined as distinct categories of mental disorders in current classification systems (ICD-10, DSM-IV-R, DSM-5), exceeds the level of random associations both in adult and paediatric populations (Caron and Rutter, 1991; Jensen, 2003). It seems, however, to be more pronounced in child and adolescent populations than in adults. In order to illustrate the impact of co-morbidities on study recruitment, a few examples will be provided. For example, ADHD in children and adolescents was found to co-occur in 52% of patients with at least one psychiatric condition and in 26.2% with two or more (Buitelaar et al., 2003; Jensen and Steinhausen, 2015). In a large European observational study with a sample size of almost 1500 (paediatric) ADHD patients (ADORE Study: Steinhausen and Novic, 2006), the following disorders were found to co-occur with ADHD: in 67% oppositional defiant disorder, in 46% a conduct disorder, in 46% anxiety disorders, and in 32% depressive disorders. Substantial amounts of overlap with other psychiatric disorders are also found in paediatric anxiety disorders, depressive disorders, and many others (Fegert and Kölch, 2011). Studies with co-morbid patients can raise a specific (sub)type regulatory question, coined by the US Food and Drug Administration (FDA) as the 'pseudospecificity issue'. This can be illustrated by the following example: When in an efficacy study, ADHD patients with co-morbid anxiety disorders are successfully treated by a drug; it is unclear whether the improvement in clinical condition was due to a (genuine) effect on ADHD or on the anxiety disorders (or on both). This is a particular issue in cases of co-morbidities where the symptom patterns of the disorders are not distinct but show some similarity or overlap. As a consequence the therapeutic claim (here: efficacy in ADHD), based on patient groups with co-morbid conditions, can be doubtful. In addition, co-morbidities tend to decrease treatment effects and result in a larger proportion of treatment resistance. Therefore study protocols exclude, as a rule, co-morbidities or do allow them only in well-defined exceptional cases. The latter include cases where a distinction between primary and secondary disorders can be fairly reliably made or where the co-morbid disorder is judged to be fairly mild and not requiring additional drug treatment. Co-morbidities, when substantial (as in the earlier case of ADHD populations), can create major risks and challenges for the successful conduct of clinical studies if they are not appropriately taken into account for study planning and in feasibility assessments. In such cases, they will result in considerable overestimations of the number of subjects available for the planned clinical trials and lead to unpleasant surprises in terms of major problems in patient recruitment and with the overall study timelines.

- *Age-specific stratifications in studies with mixed children/adolescent groups*: In a previous section of this article, it was already pointed out that for studies that plan to include both children and adolescents, it is recommendable to consider a stratification of these age groups. Stratifications are recommendable if differential response rates are likely to occur in different patient subgroups with the same clinical indications. Not controlling for factors of differential response can lead to significant fluctuations of study results from study to study (e.g. positive vs not positive study) without convincing post hoc explanations. Differential response can only be demonstrated if the sample sizes for the subgroups are sufficiently large so that there is adequate statistical power for efficacy evaluation within each of the subgroups. It was already explained that stratifications will have an impact on recruitment timelines or the number of required study sites if there are significant differences in prevalence rates between the stratified groups, and this indeed applies to children and adolescents for many clinical indications. If such differences in prevalence rates are not adequately taken into account, the recruitment of the subgroup with the lower prevalence rate is likely to considerably slow down the overall recruitment and study timelines. A strategy, which could avoid the impact of significant lower recruitment rates in children on the overall study timelines, is to have separate studies for children and adolescents. This strategy is unlikely to have an impact on the timelines of the overall paediatric development programme, but it will facilitate an earlier conclusion of studies with one of the subgroups (which in most cases will be the adolescent studies). Another advantage of separating the age groups by different studies, as opposed to mixed children/adolescent studies, is that in studies with only one age group, study sites cannot compensate their poor recruitment of children by higher recruitment rates in adolescents. If study fees for both groups are the same, it will be financially more rewarding for most sites to focus on adolescents, which will even further increase the gap between the recruitment rates for both age groups.

- *Pure drug studies* vs *studies with combined drug and psychosocial treatment*: Unless specific combination treatments are the explicit study target, they are usually avoided in clinical studies. Combination treatment cannot control for confounding factors in terms of additive or even interactive effects. Therefore efficacy studies tend to exclude the combination of the test drug with other drugs or other types of treatment (such as psychotherapies) and require an appropriate wash-out period of previous treatment in order to avoid significant carry-over effects. However, there are well-justifiable exceptions to this rule, and it is worthwhile considering these exceptions for some indications in paediatric psychiatry. Monotherapy studies and the 'wash-out' of previous treatment effects are likely to cause major feasibility issues if they are in contrast to current treatment standards that require combination treatment or consider psychotherapies/psychosocial treatment as a first-line treatment. The latter is often the case in paediatric psychiatry. The study feasibility problem will be even further enhanced if in such cases, study protocols exclude psychotherapeutic treatment within several weeks prior to study start. This not only may lead to difficult discussions with IRBs/ECs and endanger study approval but also, even if approved, will result in major recruitment difficulties. In clinical indications where psychotherapy is recommended as first-line treatment by treatment guidelines, a specific study design that takes these guidelines into consideration might be more appropriate. This would be an enrichment study with sequential study periods. Only nonresponders (or patients with insufficient response) to psychosocial treatment in the initial study period would be allowed to be randomised to placebo-controlled treatment in the subsequent double-blind study period. This is not the place for discussing the various methodological features and consequences of such study designs—for more details, see chapter on 'Study Design'. But the potential beneficial impact of such designs for patient recruitment is obvious. The caveat is that such study designs require a close ongoing monitoring of responder/nonresponder rates in the initial phase with psychosocial treatment and adaptive modifications in the required number of recruited patients. In other words, this adds another complicating factor to the planning of recruitment figures because both the initial screen failure rates plus the qualification/nonqualification rate in the initial study phase needs to be factored into the projection of randomised patients for the main study phase.
- *Requirement of contraceptive medication for female adolescents*: For most experimental drugs, potential effects on fertility and potential teratogenic effects are not yet fully assessed. Therefore the requirement of an adequate contraceptive medication in clinical trials with adolescent female patients is medically justified. In general, this does not cause a problem. But in some cultures and subcultures, mainly those with specific standards for sexual behaviour,

this may be considered a major ethical problem. In such cases, study approval is endangered or, if granted, may lead to major patient recruitment issues for female adolescent patients. Therefore it will be important to include such considerations in the selection of countries for the planned study.

- *Number of assessments per visit day*: In view of increasing study costs and in order to get as much information as possible from a study (e.g. for creating an attractive differential product profile of the new drug), clinical studies have over the last decades added an increasing number of assessments. Whereas some decades ago, psychopharmacology studies usually included, besides core safety assessments, only a primary efficacy outcome measure—usually a symptom rating scale—and, as secondary outcome measure, a clinical global rating and perhaps an additional rating of a more specific symptom dimension, current study protocols tend to foresee a list of 5–10 or sometimes even more scales. These include, besides the earlier assessments, several scales for specific symptom dimensions, sometimes both clinician ratings and patients' self-rating for the same areas; cognitive performance tests; treatment satisfaction and quality-of-life scales; health-care utilisation assessments; and sometimes also (self- and observer-) ratings of specific adverse event types (e.g. sexual functioning). There may be good justifications for each of these assessments, but, overall, the total number and time needed per visit day is often too demanding for patients and likely to have negative consequences on study quality and outcome. First, more assessments mean more frequent and lengthy investigator–patient interactions, and frequent lengthy investigator–patient interactions involve an increased risk of placebo effects. Second, lengthy assessments per visit day lead to decreases or major fluctuations in attention, as well as increased tiredness and demotivation of the study participants. It is well known from psychometric research that increases in the number of scale items and length of assessments show a curvilinear relationship with the reliability of assessments—initially, reliability tends to increase but with further assessments to considerably decrease. The issue is increased when dealing with patient populations where attention and motivation problems are part of the disorder. It is further enhanced in paediatric populations with mental disorders where disease-related attentional and motivational problems are combined with limitations associated with the cognitive and motivational developmental status. Severe effects on attention and motivation will have an impact on patient retention rates. Therefore multiple assessments that take several hours per visit days need to be avoided. In case there are convincing reasons to add assessments, multiple breaks will be necessary. It is recommendable to conduct an exploratory feasibility study in a small group of representative patients to investigate the impact of the planned assessments on patients' attention and motivation.
- *Selection of clinical raters (number of raters per site and their experience and training)*: About 20 years ago, study protocols rarely elaborated on rater selection criteria but simply stated that raters must be clinically qualified and experienced in using rating scales in the target patient group. In more recent years, protocols tend to elaborate in much more details on rater selection and qualification criteria. This trend is based on good intentions and scientific considerations to enhance the reliability and validity of clinical ratings. However, sometimes the selection criteria are too specific, and three, four, or more raters per study site are required. This tends to exclude study sites that otherwise would qualify for the study. A typical example of too specific rater selection criteria is requirements that the candidates must have worked with a specific scale in a minimum number of patients (e.g. 20 or 50) for at least 1 or 2 years. In particular, in case of newer scales and for specific symptom areas, which do not belong to the standard assessments, it is hard to meet these requirements. In addition, such specific rater selection criteria do not make sense in case of someone with

an educational background in the methodology of rating scales and experience in specific type of scales (e.g. depression rating scales) and the target patient population. People with such a background can easily transfer their experience from one scale to another similar. Sometimes, rater qualification criteria even include very questionable requirements (such as that the rater must have a 'master's degree'—in which area?). The essential selection criteria should be the following: (a) understanding the methodology of assessments (i.e. the concepts and impact of standardised assessments and scoring, reliability, and validity), (b) clinical experience with the target patient population, and (c) familiarity with the type of assessment used (e.g. a specific type of scale or test). Rater training tends to focus on correct scoring, and rater qualification is assessed by comparisons of ratings with a gold standard. An important aspect often forgotten in rater trainings and rater selection processes is interviewing skills. The reliability and validity of scorings of patient reports are a function of the precision and specificity of these reports, and these are dependent on the questions asked in the clinical interview. Therefore interviewing skills need to be an important component of rater qualifications. The impact of interviewing skills on ratings could be reduced if structured rather than semistructured clinical interviews were used. Scales with structured interviews are increasingly used in adult psychopharmacology studies, whereas their use is relatively rare in paediatric psychopharmacology studies. The construction and development of better clinical rating scales with more standardised assessment would be an important improvement for paediatric psychopharmacology studies. Less structured interviews have a lower reliability (and validity) than structured interviews, and lower reliabilities of assessments require larger sample sizes to demonstrate statistically significant treatment effects.
- Size and number of the investigational product (IP): Especially, children are likely to have difficulties in swallowing capsules of a bigger size or several capsules simultaneously. If this is not taken care of in the manufacturing of the IP and parents/caregivers do not regularly control the intake of the IP, this can result in major medication compliance issues and have a negative impact on study results.

10.8 Specific aspects of study monitoring

Study monitoring plays an important role in ensuring and securing data quality. Both clinical research assistants and medical monitors will be needed for these tasks. Monitoring includes the following:

(a) Checking the completeness of the data provided in the case record forms (CRFs).
(b) Source data checking (in medical records) to confirm the verifiability and accuracy of data provided in the CRFs.
(c) Ensuring adherence to study protocol requirements (patient selection criteria and other protocol regulations such as time and sequence of assessments).
(d) Plausibility checks in terms of cross-checking of data from different assessments (e.g. diagnosis, co-morbidity and concomitant medication, and adverse events) to become aware of possible inconsistencies in the information provided.

Close collaborations between site monitors and medical monitors will be necessary to achieve high data quality and validity of the study data. In the following, some specific aspects of study monitoring have been selected that can help overcoming issues and hurdles in patient recruitment and study conduct and are helpful in enhancing the quality of efficacy data coming from clinical rating scales:

- *Monitoring patient recruitment and study conduct challenges*: It is important to carefully monitor issues and hurdles in patient recruitment and study conduct, discuss them with the study sites, and bring them to the attention of study management. In some cases, it will be sufficient to better explain protocol requirements to the study sites; in others, it could be useful to organise small investigator meetings (e.g. telephone conferences) to provide opportunities for an exchange of experience (questions: Do other study sites have the same issues? How do they manage to overcome them?). It is not recommendable to invite for those meetings only sites that are having difficulties. This could increase the risk of ending up in nothing but a list of difficulties, which may further demotivate many investigators. Therefore the participation of investigators that are well recruiting and experienced in paediatric psychopharmacology trials will be essential for such meetings to be successful. These investigators could provide advice on how to overcome certain issues. They can also help to identify issues that are indeed related to unrealistic study-specific requirements and may need additional support measures or even require modifications of study protocol features. The availability of electronic CRFs will allow ongoing real-time inspections and reviews of recruitment data and repeated evaluations throughout the study for different levels—the study, country, and site level. This enables a quick identification of recruitment and timeline issues, identifies sites that need special attention and support, and can also provide feedback on the impact of specific training and support measures.
- *Monitoring of possible rating trends and biases*: In addition, such electronic systems could be used to become aware of trends and biases in efficacy ratings and to reveal differences in rater trends between sites and countries. This could be done without unblinding treatment allocations. This type of monitoring would help to identify 'critical' sites and countries, which show 'unusual' ratings that differ from most of the other sites. It also would allow early implementations of corrective measures, for example, additional training and instructions. A few examples will help to illustrate this point:
  - Example 1: Study sites may differ in the type of recruited patients. One group of sites may, for example, almost exclusively recruit patients with fairly mild degrees of disease severity; others may have a majority of patients with high degrees of severities; and the third group may recruit patients, which represent the entire spectrum of severity. None of these sites may have violated any protocol requirements, but marked differences in baseline severity between sites may lead to different types of rater habits and biases. The selection of only mildly ill patients is, for example, likely to increase placebo responder rates. In case of a highly selective recruitment strategy, it would be necessary to better understand the underlying reasons and consider how to help sites to recruit a broader spectrum of patients (e.g. by considering different types of patient referral systems).
  - Example 2: Similarly, ongoing (blinded!) evaluations of ratings could indicate that at some sites or countries, the number of patients with significant improvements exceeds by far the proportion of improvements expected from a 1:1 randomisation to active drug or placebo. This would raise suspicions that part of these patients was most likely placebo responders.
  - Example 3: Ongoing evaluations could also draw attention to patients with dramatic changes in their efficacy ratings from one postbaseline assessment day to the next—or with drastic discrepancies between ratings in scales that are known to measure similar types of behaviour or symptoms.

The suggested monitoring of ratings is not intended to correct efficacy results by replacing them with other ratings. It is rather used to increase awareness of possible rater trends and biases and to provide early additional specific training.

10.9 Conclusion

This chapter describes various study management tasks and challenges related to the planning, implementation, and conduct of clinical drug studies in paediatric psychopharmacology. Not all such tasks were discussed but only those with particular relevance for a successful study conduct and outcome. Clinical studies are scientific projects, which is why their top priority must be the quality of the generated data. In scientific terms, this means that the studies must have an adequate internal and external validity to be able to address the defined primary and secondary study questions. Methodologically and clinically adequate study protocols have a prominent role in ensuring good data quality. But protocols are only plans. The produced data quality will finally depend on how study protocols are executed, and this highlights the important role of operational processes, monitoring, and study management. In addition, not all good plans are necessarily feasible within a realistic timeframe and in consideration of the financial and manpower resources available.

The description and discussion of various tasks and challenges related to the setup, implementation, and running of clinical studies has illustrated and demonstrated the importance of study operations and management for successful clinical studies. However, this discussion also demonstrated that in order to achieve high quality data, operational planning and solutions need to be adequately informed. They require a background of good scientific methodological and medical understanding and knowledge of the study population, the assessment methods, and the experimental designs. In case of paediatric psychopharmacology studies, this involves knowledge of and experience with mental disorders in children and adolescents, available treatment options, paediatric efficacy scales, and implications of specific study designs (e.g. placebo-controlled studies). Without such background knowledge and experience, a majority of study challenges cannot be adequately understood and addressed, and there will be the risk of wrong decisions, that is, decisions that are likely to affect the quality and validity of study data. On the other hand, in order to make studies feasible, medical scientists and specialists need to sufficiently understand the operational consequences of protocol requirements and must be willing to discuss them and listen to possible concerns of their operational colleagues.

On top of challenges associated with almost all types of clinical studies, paediatric psychopharmacology studies involve some specific challenges to clinical researchers and study management. Study approval and patient recruitment appears to be often more challenging than for adult studies. Special legal conditions will apply. Study procedures and assessment methods and schedules have to take the developmental status of the clinical trial subjects into account. Standard study designs known from adult studies may have to be modified in order to adjust to paediatric indications. Finally, as demonstrated in another chapter of this book, placebo responder rates tend to be significantly higher in paediatric populations than in adults, which is a big challenge for efficacy studies in paediatric psychopharmacology that needs a good understanding and adequate handling.

References

American Academy of Child and Adolescent Psychiatry, 1998. Practice parameters for the assessment and treatment of children and adolescents with depressive disorders. J. Am. Acad. Child Adolesc. Psychiatry 37 (Suppl), 63S–83S.

Bridge, J.A., Birmaher, B., Iyengar, S., Barbe, R.P., Brent, D.A., 2009. Placebo response in randomized controlled trials of antidepressants for pediatric major depressive disorder. Am. J. Psychiatry 166, 42–49.

Buitelaar, J.K., Montgomery, S.A., van Zwieten-Boot, B.J., 2003. Attention deficit hyperactivity disorder: guidelines for investigating efficacy of pharmacological intervention. Eur. Neuropsychopharmacol. 13, 297–304.

Caron, C., Rutter, M., 1991. Comorbidity in child psychopharmacology: concepts, issues and research strategies. J. Child Psychol. Psychiatry 32 (7), 1063–1080.

Emslie, G.J., Heiligenstein, J.H., Wagner, K.D., Hoog, S.L., Ernest, D.E., Brown, E., Nilsson, M., Jacobson, J.G., 2002. Fluoxetine for acute treatment of depression in children and adolescents: a placebo-controlled, randomized clinical trial. J. Am. Acad. Child Adolesc. Psychiatr. 41 (10), 1205–1215.

Fegert, J.M., Kölch, M., 2011. Klinikmanual Kinder- und Jugendpsychiatrie und –psychotherapie. Springer, Berlin, Heidelberg.

Jensen, C.M., 2003. Comorbidity and child psychopathology. Recommendations for the next decade. J. Abnorm. Child Psychol. 31 (3), 293–300.

Jensen, C.M., Steinhausen, H.C., 2015. Comorbid mental disorders in children and adolescents with attention deficit/hyperactivity disorder in a large nationwide study. Atten. Deficit Hyperact. Disord. 7, 27–38.

Khan, A., Brown, W., 2015. Antidepressant versus placebo in major depression: an overview. World Psychiatry 14, 294–300.

Khan, A., Mar, K.F., Faucett, J., Khan Shilling, S., Brown, W.A., 2017. Has the rising placebo response impacted antidepressant clinical trial outcome? Data from the US Food and Drug Administration 1987-2013. World Psychiatry 16 (2), 181–192.

Levine, R.J., 1988. Ethics and Regulation in Clinical Research. Yale University Press, New Haven, London.

Levy, M.D.L., Larcher, V., Kurz, R., the members of the Ethics Working Group of the CESP, 2003. Informed consent/assent in children. Statement of the Ethics Working Group of the Confederation of European Specialists in Paediatrics (CESP). Eur. J. Pediatr. 162, 629–633.

Rutherford, B.R., Roose, S.P., 2013. A model of placebo response in antidepressant clinical trials. Am. J. Psychiatry 170 (7), 723–733. http://10.1176/appi.ajp.2012.12040474.

Steinhausen, H.C., Novic, T.C., the ADORE Study Group, 2006. Coexisting psychiatric problems in ADHD in the ADORE cohort. Eur. Child Adolesc. Psychiatry 15 (1), 1125–1170.

Walsh, B.T., Seidman, S.N., Sysko, R., Gould, M., 2002. Placebo response in studies with major depression: variable, substantial, and growing. JAMA 287 (14), 1840–1847.

Listening to the patients' voice

Deborah Lee
AlaWai Neurology Consulting LLC, Honolulu, HI, United States

11.1 Introduction

In the development of new medications, the patient/caregiver perspective plays an increasingly critical role. This chapter will explore ways this perspective is being solicited, how different players in the drug development arena are using this information, and how in some cases patient/caregivers are changing laws to drive their agendas. The objectives of this chapter will consist of the following (Table 11.1)

(a) to review different methods by which information from patients' and caregivers can be solicited;
(b) to review how regulatory agencies are incorporating the patient/caregivers' voice in all aspects of drug development including drug approvals;
(c) to review how patient advocacy groups are shaping the future of academic research;
(d) to review how payers are incorporating the patient/caregivers' opinion in reimbursement decisions and how patient advocacy groups can fight back;
(e) to review how patients are taking the matter of drug availability into their own hands with legislation;
(f) to present an example: two essays provided by a patient with autism, the first as a child, aged 7, and the second as an adult.

11.2 Soliciting patient/caregiver/caregiver perspective

There are multiple methods for interested parties to solicit information from patients/caregivers. Interested parties such as regulatory agencies, academic centres, and pharmaceutical groups may form partnerships with patient/caregiver advocacy organisations. Often, this means that one or two elected advocates represent the entire group. These representatives are invited to speak at FDA Advisory Committees, providing input into development programmes, and even have active membership in clinical trial steering committees.

Another method of obtaining information is to work with advocacy groups to design patient/caregiver surveys which will be sent to registered members. The information may be particularly beneficial in cases where there isn't sufficient information in the literature focusing a certain aspect of the disease or a patient/caregiver viewpoint is needed regarding determining most important targets for drug intervention. One example was a web-based survey sponsored by the Reflex Sympathetic Dystrophy Syndrome Association (RSDSA) that provided significant insight into patient perspective on coping with this serious disease (Sharma et al., 2009). Results of these surveys may be provided to regulatory agencies.

Table 11.1 Key points to remember in listening to the patients' voice

• Incorporating the patients/caregivers' voice is critical to drug development
• Patient information can be solicited in multiple different ways:
• through patient advocacy groups
• through patient surveys
• through participation in protocol steering committees
• Regulatory agencies and payer groups are soliciting advice from patient groups with regard to drug approval, protocol design, and reimbursement
• It is important to include clinicians in these conversations to improve clarity around patient/caregiver input
• How best to maximise incorporation of the patient/caregiver viewpoint is still evolving

There are also formal websites, often covering multiple disorders, where patient/caregivers may enter their data which then may be accessed by other groups such as pharmaceutical companies. One example is Patients Like Me. In addition to patient/caregiver advocacy groups that tend to be often disease specific, there are disease-independent organisations that act on behalf of patient/caregivers in interactions with pharmaceutical companies and regulatory agencies and support clinical trials such as National Organization for Rare Disorders (NORD) and ICAN. Also, note that these activities are not restricted to adults. The Young Persons' Advisory Group (YPAG) is an organisation composed of youths who provide advice to researchers regarding their development plans and programmes.

Finally, patient/caregiver advocacy groups can be crucial in supporting enrolment for clinical trials, especially in rare disorders.

The following sections will describe the four critical avenues for patient/caregiver participation in the United States: regulatory agencies, academic societies, pharmaceutical companies, and health technology assessments by payers.

11.3 Regulatory agencies (FDA)

The FDA has been soliciting patient/caregiver input via the Patient Representative Program since 1991. This programme has strict criteria for patient/caregiver representatives and a standardised application process and provides training. Once selected, these patient/caregiver representatives serve as special government employees (SGE) providing patient/caregiver perspective into clinical trials and postapproval phases of medicinal product development. In addition, they are voting members of product advisory committees and can influence whether a product is approved (FDA: Advisory Committees: Critical to the FDA's Product Review Process).

This participation has been expanded in the Food and Drug Administration Act (FDASIA) Section 1137 which states

(a) IN GENERAL. The secretary shall develop and implement strategies to solicit the views of patients during the medical product development process and consider the perspectives of patient/caregivers during regulatory discussions, including by

(1) fostering participation of a patient representative who may serve as a special government employee in appropriate agency meetings with medical product sponsors and investigators; and
(2) exploring means to provide for identification of patient representatives who do not have any, or have minimal, financial interests in the medical products industry.

Participation of patient/caregiver representatives is especially important where FDA may have concerns about the strength of the data or the level of risk; patient/caregiver representatives may advocate for approval, especially in cases where there is an unmet clinical need and/or life-threatening diseases. This strong advocacy can even lead to changes in FDA approval process such as the development of an accelerated approval pathway after the significant input from the HIV population (Edgar and Rothman, 1990).

Patient/caregiver groups have been involved in writing draft FDA guidance for conduction of studies. One example is the draft guidance for indication studies in muscular dystrophy written by the Parent Project Muscular Dystrophy Transcript: Director's Corner-Working with patient advocacy groups. In it, they suggested that the current practice of using the 6-min walk test as a primary endpoint excluded nonambulatory patients from participating and that these patients may also benefit from drugs in development. This guidance entitled 'Duchenne Muscular Dystrophy: Developing Drugs for Treatment over the Spectrum of Disease' was submitted to FDA on 26 June 2014 and is currently undergoing review (Furlong et al., 2015).

Patient/caregiver input is not limited to drugs; FDA also has guidance regarding patient input into devices as well (FDA).

While information from patient/caregivers has been sought since 1990, recently gaps have been identified comparing what FDA expects and what patient/caregiver groups are able to provide. One of the greatest challenges for patient/caregiver groups is how to transform patient/caregiver experience data from anecdotes into clinically meaningful, empirical endpoints. While FDA is willing to accept data from patient/caregivers, it expects that it will have the same level of rigour as nonpatient/caregiver data. This is often a block for patient/caregiver advocacy groups as they do not have the resources that will be required to obtain these data (Kuehn, 2018).

Currently, there is a strong movement to expand access to nonapproved drugs outside of clinical trials. One example was the expanded access programme for Epidiolex (a synthetic cannabidiol) in children with refractory epilepsy (Throckmorton, 2014).

While the European Medicines Agency (EMA) has not formalised a procedure by which patient/caregivers can influence drug development, there is indication that interest exists. A presentation by Andrea Furia-Helms on patient/caregiver involvement at FDA can be found on the EMA website, and there exists several public declarations of interests and confidentiality undertaking of European Medicines Agency from patient/caregivers who act as consultants in European-focused pharmaceutical companies and declaring interest to act as experts for the EMA. However, an initial call by the European Commission in September 2011 for a 'civil society' representation from patient/caregivers resulted in a low number of applications, and the call was relaunched in July 2012. In addition, the more rigid privacy laws that exist in Europe compared with the United States may play a role, and the more recent experience in human experimentation that took place last century may influence the willingness of patient/caregivers to engage companies and regulatory agencies.

11.4 Academic associations

Patient/caregivers are a driving force for drug development through participation in medical societies and their own fund-raising efforts. Oftentimes, patient/caregiver groups are included in discussions regarding appropriate trial designs. For example, American Academy of Child and Adolescent Psychiatry in collaboration with Best Practice invited patient/caregiver representatives to participate in the development of a consensus report (Carson et al., 2003) where it was recommended that parents of children with the disorder being studied should be included on pharmaceutical companies' advisory boards.

This is especially true with rare diseases where patient/caregiver advocacy groups have increased public awareness including public, media, and legislative interest in rare diseases. These groups have been involved in helping patient/caregiver recruitment and review of protocol design (Groft, 2013). Mechanisms are being developed to measure caregivers/patients' preferences for treatment and acceptability of risks (Peay et al. 2014)

Patient advocacy groups are also participating in significant fund-raising efforts. In this way, they can have a direct influence on current research, especially early phases (Litterman et al. 2014).

11.5 Pharmaceutical companies

There has been an increasing level of involvement of patient/caregiver advocacy groups in pharmaceutical company-sponsored drug development, dependent on the groups' resources, expertise, and priorities. This involvement can include generating FDA Guidance for Industry documents outlining important critical factors in developing safe and effective drugs (see Parent Project Muscular Dystrophy earlier). Even smaller groups that might lack sufficient resources and expertise required for direct investment in drug development can sponsor clinical trial networks that take an active part in increasing awareness of clinical trials, identifying appropriate trial candidates, expediting patient/caregiver enrolment, and improving site efficiency (Rose et al., 2015). This is especially important for drug development in rare diseases where it may be difficult to enrol patient/caregivers at local sites without an extensive network.

In addition, more and more pharmaceutical companies are soliciting advice from patient advocacy groups in all aspects of protocol design. This may range from caregiver acceptability of blood sampling for pharmacokinetic studies in a paediatric population to the design of patient/caregiver friendly reported outcome measures such as seizure diaries for epilepsy trials.

When working with patient advocacy groups, it is important to assess the level of experience that the group has with clinical trial development. This is especially important in managing expectations. Advocacy groups often like to be involved early in the development process, and the more experienced patient advocacy groups understand that often programmes they have consulted on do not move forwards for various reasons. They just want to be informed early when such programmes are terminated and for whatever reasons that can be shared publicly. Care should be taken in educating less mature/experienced advocacy groups that their involvement does not guarantee that the programme will be completed. Full transparency should always be the goal in any relationship with patient advocacy groups. It is also advisable that, if possible, clinicians with experience in treating patient/caregivers be a part of any discussion with patient advocacy groups. They can provide significant insight between what patient/caregivers say and what they mean.

In September 2017, the European Federation of Pharmaceutical Industries and Associations (EFPIA) published an interesting document named 'Working together with patient groups'. This document was cocreated by the representatives of patient organisations and the research-based pharmaceutical industry through the EFPIA Patient Think Tank. If the aim of the document, underlining the rationale for interactions between the pharmaceutical industry and patient organisations and suggesting the key principles of collaboration, is quite informative, the thought process that drove the inception of such think tank illustrates well the current and necessary changes in drug development. Information on the EFPIA Patient Think Tank can be found at www.efpia.eu/relationships-codes/patient-organisations/the-patient-think-tank/.

11.6 Payer groups (health technology assessments)

Even after a drug is approved, there is often a separate review, known as health technology assessments, to determine if the drug should be covered by insurance companies or government agencies. Patient/caregivers have become more involved in these discussions, but the same with FDA and drug approvals, there are discussions on what does meaningful patient/caregiver input look like. Rozmovits et al. (2018) in examining the pan-Canadian Oncology Drug Review noted that 'There is a fundamental tension between the evidence-based nature of health technology assessments and the experientially oriented culture of patient/caregiver advocacy'. They noted that good practices for incorporating patient/caregiver information included (1) engagement with patient/caregivers early; (2) engagement of a range of patient/caregivers; (3) leverage patient-provided information, data resources, and outreach mechanisms; (4) transparency; and (5) appreciation and accommodation of resource constraints (Perfetto et al., 2018). And patient/caregivers are leveraging their voices if insurance companies are denying treatment that they feel should be reimbursed; a good example is the Parent Project Muscular Dystrophy organisation (Ionita et al., 2018).

11.7 Patients: Direct to legislation

In the United States, if patient/caregivers feel that they are not being heard or being denied what they are owed, they may also resort to legislation. Two examples include the right-to-try law which has been enacted by 40 states. The law basically states that terminally ill patients have the right to experimental therapies that have completed Phase 1 testing but have not been approved by FDA. Currently, since the law does not obligate the pharmaceutical companies to provide the drug or for payers to pay for the drug, the current law may have limited value; however, that may change in the future as advocacy groups become more militant. Another example is the access to medical marijuana while still illegal at the US federal level has been legalised in 29 states as of 2018.

11.7.1 The patient's voice

Below are two essays written by Chance first as a child, aged 7, and second as an adult. He was tasked with the assignment of teaching other children about what it is like to have autism. These essays are excerpts taken from a guidebook for children with neurological diseases which included essays by the children themselves (Lee, 2015).

11.7.2 Chance (age 7)

> My name is Chance, I am seven years old and I have autism. I do not understand what this is, but I do know that it makes me different from others. I like playing with trains, riding bikes and playing video games. My favorite game is Pokemon because I really like the way the characters evolve into other forms. I think I am very good at my game boy color. I have a love for books and learned how to read since the age of two. I want to be a meteorologist when I grow up and have read many books on this subject. My mom always tells me that just because I have autism doesn't mean I can't be anything I want to be when I grow up.
> Because I am different I don't have many friends. It's not that I don't want to make friends, but I don't understand how to make friends. Everyone should have a friend, just because I have a different way of doing things doesn't mean that I can't be a good friend. I don't like many types of foods, they feel weird on my tongue and taste yucky. My favorites are plain rice, slice bread, cereal (no milk) and of course a plain cheeseburger from McDonald's. In the first grade I was in the school play and was chosen to sing the music solo, I liked that a lot.
> I am now in second grade. I am in a regular classroom with everyone else so I don't feel so different there. I really love school and think I am smart. I make the honor roll and study hard. I was chosen to be in the school spelling bee.
> Riding bikes is my favorite past time. Dr. Lee tells me you should always wear your helmet when riding a bike, so I do. I have a lot of pets like my too fish, one dog and seven cats that I love to spend time with. We are four people in my family my dad, mom, older sister and myself. I love my family, I know my family loves me and they do not treat me any different because I have autism. Autism is not like other disabilities. You cannot tell I have this just by looking at me. I am different and that's ok because remember God made each and every one of us in his likeness even though we may be different to the world.

11.7.3 Chance (adult)

I had looked at the essay that Dr. Lee sent me before I wrote this follow-up essay, and I was amazed at how much had changed in roughly fourteen years. After all, life is full of changes. However, that does not mean that everything has changed- at least, not fully or more completely than not- but life does, indeed, have its changes. One can say that at least one of the purposes of writing this follow-up essay was to respond to the one that I had written when I was seven. I have certainly come a long way since then. Autism makes me different mainly in the way that I communicate and process, and I did come to realize that, at least more and more, sometime as I matured. However, I do not believe that anyone- other than God- can ever fully understand autism, myself included. Autism is a part ofe me; I live with it, I accept it, and I do not fully understand it, but it does not have to define me. Rather, I let the fact that I am a perfect child in the eyes of God define me. Continuing on the subject of activities, hobbies, and whatnot, unless you count video games- which I have liked playing for at least most of my life, at least up to the point of when I completed this essay, and likely do still like playing-involving them or something along those linesor if I do so with a friend, with a relative, or whatnot for whatever reason, I do not play with trains or ride bikes anymore. I also do not like Pokémon anymore. As for reading, although I do not have nearly as much time as I used to for reading, I still like to do so. Although I no longer want to be a meteorologist, as I did when I was seven, I have always had- and likely still do have-an interest in weather- and natural disaster-related things. Finally, in response to the last statement in the first paragraph of the essay that I worte when I was seven, it is true that just because one has autsim does not mean- at least when it comes to one's calling, I believe, anyway- that he or she cannot be anything that he or she wants to be when he or she grows up. When it comes to accomplishing things, autism is not necessarily an impenetrable wall, but rather, an obstacle that has to be overcome. When autism is indeed an obstacle, it can indeed bt overcome.

Continuing in a similar vein, just because one is different does not mean that one cannot have many friends. Although I am still working on making friends, talking to people, strengthening relationships, and whatnot- all of these require continuous work, of course- I certainly have more friends than when I was seven. Friendship can be difficult to understand, at least at times, but I have picked up more understanding about it. I believe that everyone should have several friends. It does not matter if you do different things or do things differently when it comes to being a good friend; anyone can do it. I also believe that you do, however, have to choose your frinds wisely, especially when ti comes to closer and closer friends. When it comes to food, I have certainly expanded my horizon; I now like many types of food, my favorites at the time of writing this essay being potato salad-without relish- jambalaya, fried butterfly shrimp, and perhaps others that I have left out. I also like some fruits such as bananas, blueberries, and, perhaps my favorite lind of fruit, raspberries, although my horizon certainly is not limited to the things that I have listed, although I do still like plain rice, sliced bread, cereal without milk-although when I eat it, I eat ti with milk at least most of the time now- and plain cheeseburgers from McDonald's. As for the school play in the first grade, I honestly do not remember singing a solo, although I do remember, among other things, that it was a Christmas-related play and that I was one of the three kings bringing gifts to Jesus.

I began writing this essay when I was a junior at the University of Louisiana at Lafayette, and I completed it somewhat shortly after becoming a senior. A times, at least, I have felt that I was at least somewhat busy to the point of not working on the essay, at least, very often to at least some degree and- or alternatively, or- quickly to at least some degree. I have always been in regular classrooms, but notably, I took special keyboarding and handwriting-and whatnot, perhaps, which I have mentioned because I do not quite remember- sessions in elementary school and study skills classes throughout middle school and high school, and additionally- at least, again, at the time of writing this- I was enrolled in the Office of Disability Services and the Student Support Services programs at UL Lafayette. I believe that they have helped me significantly in my education. Like when I was seven and whatnot, in the regular classrooms, I have not felt so different, and additionally- again, like when I was seven and whatnot- I have liked school. I believe God has blessed me with wisdom and intelligence. To, I believe, at least some degree of notability, I have achieved a 4.0\GPA in high school, and additionally- again, at least at the time of writing this- I have kept a 4.0 GPA at UL Lafayette. Other than once if the fifth grade, I have made the honor roll- and, I believe, the principal's list at times- throughout elementary school and middle school. As for the spelling bee, I was a participant in a spelling be when I was in first grade; I believe I made it to the top three, but I lost when I misspelled the word "straight." "S-t-r-a-i-t," I believe, was the way that I spelled it; my late grandmother- on my mom's side of the family- got me a trophy, though. In one's life, there are ups and downs as well as vicoties and defeats, and I believe that most if not all people experience each- or a combination- of these at least once in life.

I have not ridden a bike in years, although I may ride again in the future. However, for one to wear a helmet when riding a bike is, I believe, good advice! As for pets, at least at the time of completing this, I had- about, at least- five guppies-fancy guppies, I believe- a small catfish- a cory, or perhaps Cory, catfish, I believe, but at least at the time of writing this essay, I did not remember if it is called a striped cory catfish, a spotted cory catfish, or whatnot-an aquatic tiger nerite snail, and a snapping turtle as pets. I like my pets. I am still in a family of four, but at the time of writing this, I have not lived with my sister for years, though I have still seen her at times. I still love my family, and I always will. My family still loves me, and I do not believe that there are very many, if any, differences in how I am treated due at least in part to me having autism. In response to the third- and second-to-last statements in the essay that I wrote when I was seven, I believe that autism is not like, at least, many other disabilities ans that it is at least somewhat difficult to tell that I have autism by looking at me. In response to the final statement of the essay that I worte whe I was seven, I still believe that it is okay to be different. I believe that it is okay for me as well as anyone and-or alternatively, or- everyone else to be different, though. I still believe that God, despite us being different to the world- I do not quite remember if, in that last statement in the essay that I wrote when I was seven, I meant "us" and "the world" either in the context of disabilities or in the context of what might call religious beliefs, but whatever it may have been, in the writing of this essay, I intended to make this statement in the context of my beliefs-made all of us in His likeness.

I wanted to clonclude this follow-up essay with some additional information. For the work that I will have done during the course of my life, I will use the pen name- and, or alternatively, or, the nickname- C.K. Bourgeois. At least at the time of writing this essay, I was a Moving Image Arts major-that is, I primarily studies movie-making- and an English minor at UL Lafayette. I was living in Lafayette- or, perhaps, Scott, perhaps depending on how one views it- in Loiusiana. My favorite band was- and likely still is- Fireflight, and my favorite video game was- and,again, likel still is- Kirby Super Star Ultra. Besides the Bible, my favorite book, or book series- in the *case of my favorite book or book series other than the Bible, I won theentire series compiled into one book- is perhaps- and, perhaps, likely still is- The Chronocles of Narnia by C.S. Lewis. I have worked at least two jobs; one was as an usher at one of the twoGrand Theater- or, perhaps, Theatre- locations in Lafayette and the other was as an audio and, primarily, video editor in TFC Media at The Family Church in Lafayette. Finally, God has called me to be a director and a writer, and I intend, during the course of my life, to have done what I have been called to do.*

11.8 Conclusion

This chapter focussed on listening to the patients' voices in drug development. Previously the practice of medicine was very paternalistic. The physician would dictate the medical care, and patients would follow the doctor's orders without question. However, over the past few decades, patients have become more involved in interrogating the medical establishment and have taken on a more active role in determining their own care. This involvement has now expanded beyond their own care to all aspects of clinical drug development from funding research they feel is necessary to working with regulatory agencies and payers to advocate for drug approvals and reimbursement. In some cases, patients have bypassed pharmaceutical companies and regulatory agencies to create legislation to advance drug availability.

With the advent of personalised medicine, the voice of the patient/caregiver is becoming more and more critical in drug development, approval, and accessibility. It is important that regulators, academic centres, pharmaceutical companies, and payers learn to listen.

References

Carson, G.A., Jensen, P.S., Findling, R.L., Meyer, R.E., Calabrese, J., DelBello, M.P., Emslie, G., et al., 2003. Methodological issues and controversies in clinical trials with child and adolescent patient/caregivers with bipolar disorder: report of a consensus conference. J. Child Adolesc. Psychopharmacol. 13, 13–27.

Edgar, H., Rothman, D.J., 1990. New rules for new drugs: the challenge of AIDs to the regulatory process. Milbank Q. 68 (Suppl. 1), 111–142.

Furlong, P., Bridges, J.F.P., Charnas, L., Fallon, J.R., Fischer, R., Flanigan, K.M., Franson, T.R., Gulati, N., McDonald, C., Peay, H., Sweeney, H.L., 2015. How a patient/caregiver advocacy group developed the first proposed draft guidance document for industry for submission to the U.S. Food and Drug Administration. Orphanet J. Rare Dis. 10, 82.

Groft, S.C., 2013. Rare disease research: expanding collaborative translational research opportunities. Chest 144, 16–23.

Ionita, C., Kinnett, M., et al., 2018. Collective statement regarding patient access to approved therapies from the center directors of Parent Project Muscular Dystrophy's certified Duchenne Care Centers. PLoS Curr. 10. pii: ecurrents.md.4a12c57a46a24603cb3d36d7f e0668b6.

Kuehn, C.M., 2018. Patient/caregiver experience data in US Food and Drug Administration (FDA) regulatory decision making: a policy process perspective. Ther. Innov. Regul. Sci. https://doi.org/10.1177/2168479017753390. Tirs.sagepub.com.

Lee, D., 2015. Is My Brain Bocken? Xlibris.

Litterman, N.K., Rhee, M., Swinney, D.C., Ekins, S., 2014. Collaboration for rare disease drug discovery. F1000Res. 3, 261.

Peay, H.L., Hollin, I., Fischer, R., Bridges, J.F.P., 2014. A community-engaged approach to quantifying caregiver preferences for the benefits and risks of emerging therapies for Duchenne Muscular Dystrophy. Clin. Ther. 36, 624–637.

Perfetto, E.M., Harris, J., Mullins, C.D., dosReis, S., 2018. Emerging good practices for transforming value assessment: patients' voices, patient/caregivers' values. Value Health 21, 386–393.

Rose, D.M., Marshall, R., Surber, M.W., 2015. Pharmaceutical industry, academia and patient/caregiver advocacy organizations: what is the recipe for synergic (win-win-win) collaborations? Respirology 20, 185–191.

Rozmovits, L., Mai, H., Chambers, A., Chan, K., 2018. What does meaningful look like? A qualitative study of patient/caregiver engagement at the Pan-Canadian Oncology Drug-Review: perspectives of reviewers and payers. J. Health Serv. Res. Policy 23, 72–79.

Sharma, A., et al., 2009. A web-based cross-sectional epidemiological survey of complex regional pain syndrome. Reg. Anesth. Pain Med. 34, 110–115.

Throckmorton, D.C., 2014. Mixed Signals: The Administration's policy on marijuana-part four-the health effects and science. http://www.fda.gov/newsevents/testimimony/ucm402061.htm.

Further reading

European Federation of Pharmaceutical Industries and Associations (Efpia), https://www.efpia.eu/media/288492/working-together-with-patient-groups-23102017.pdf.

Food and Drug Administration, Advisory Committees: Critical to the FDA's Product Review Process. http://www.fda.gov/drugs/resourcesforyou/consumers/ucm143538.htm.

Food and Drug Administration, Transcript: Director's Corner-Working with patient advocacy groups. http://www.fda.gov/drugs/newsevents/ucm458746.htm.

Food and Drug Administration, Patient Preference Information – Voluntary Submission, Review in Premarket Approval Applications, Humanitarian Device Exemption Applications, and De Novo Requests, and Inclusion in Decision Summaries and Device Labeling. https://www.fda.gov/downloads/medicaldevices/deviceregulationandguidance/guidancedocuments/ucm446680.pdf.

Food and Drug Administration. FDASIA, http://www.fda.gov/regulatoryinformation/legislation/significantamendmentstothefdcact/fdasia/ucm311045.htm.

Furia-Helms, A., http://www.ema.europa.eu/docs/en_GB/document_library/Presentation/2015/08/WC500191864.pdf.

ICAN, https://icanresearch.org/.

National Organization Rare Disorders, https://rarediseases.org/.

Patients Like Me, https://www.patientlikeme.com/?utm_source=googlesearch&utm_medium=cpc&utm_campaign=brand_general_search_adgroup_brandedexact_lp1_h58_h57_copy58&campaignid=876379635&adgroupid=44435588552&adid=218543155100.

Young Persons Advisory Group, http://ypag.grip-network.org/.

Specificities of safety management in paediatric psychopharmacological research

Jelena Ivkovic
Early Psychiatry Projects, H. Lundbeck A/S, Copenhagen, Denmark

12.1 Introduction

Participation of children in clinical researches has been always associated with controversial connotation, mainly due to ethical aspects and challenges related to safety and tolerability. As a result, none or very limited information has been made available for use of medicine in paediatric population. To provide better treatment options for minors, the overall climate changed, and more paediatric clinical studies have been conducted over the last 10 years, providing valuable information on both efficacy and safety.

There are many aspects related to safe use of the drug in children, including meaningful and adequate assessment of safety and tolerability in preapproval phase and in postmarketing settings. An early initiation of paediatric development programme has become a must for all new compounds for which there is a potential for paediatric use. This has opened new perspectives for paediatric treatments, but it has also brought new challenges and obstacles related to participation of children in clinical studies. This chapter focuses on safety-related aspects in paediatric clinical studies, with focus on psychopharmacological research.

12.2 General considerations

Labelling information for the majority of drugs approved for human use includes none or insufficient information on safety experience in children, precise effective and safe dosing regimen, except for drugs that were developed exclusively for paediatric indications. This situation mainly results from an insufficient inclusion of paediatric populations in clinical development programmes for the vast majority of drugs. A small number of paediatric patients involved do not provide sufficient sample size for the detection of adverse drug reactions to the same degree as for adults. Rare adverse drug reactions (ADRs) can only usually be detected randomly because small sample size will limit to observe anything less than common during clinical development programme.

Therefore, to protect children from unknowns and uncertainties, the dominating thought process was to 'protect' paediatric patients from research as well. Over the last decade, fortunately, there was a gradual shift in the general paradigm of drug development in paediatric population, since newly approved drugs offer great benefit and better treatment options for them. The overall design of clinical development programmes started to expand and broaden to include different subpopulation. As a consequence of the evolvement within regulatory environment and requirements, which changed substantially over recent years, if there is a possibility that a drug can be used off-label in children, such use needs to be explored and addressed in preapproval phase rather than in postmarketing setting. Like for adult population, both efficacy and safety aspects must be thoroughly addressed and confirmed in clinical trial settings.

While investigating the efficacy of the drug in children is usually the primary objective of phase II and III studies, investigation of safety and tolerability remains another critical and challenging aspect. Safety monitoring in clinical studies is a well-regulated area by international guidelines and directives, regardless of therapeutic area or target population. Paediatric population is, however, more vulnerable in many aspects. Consequently, safety monitoring in paediatric clinical studies should be carefully and thoroughly planned and executed.

12.3 Investigating safety and tolerability in paediatric clinical trials, points to consider

All elements of safety monitoring should be based on the totality of data made available in preclinical and clinical studies and gaps that remained to be covered.

Data from preclinical studies can identify target organ toxicity and provide appropriate margins of safety between therapeutic exposure and those that produce adversity in nonclinical studies. Juvenile animal studies are an extension of this paradigm in providing a comparison between adults and immature forms of the animal species. Juvenile toxicology studies in animals provide robust and useful information for initial set-up of safety monitoring (Sheth, 2009). Toxicological studies in juvenile animals should address long-term follow-up on skeletal, neural, behavioural, sexual, and immunological maturation and development to the most considerable extent (WHO, 2007).

Safety data generated in adult population can be extrapolated to children to a certain extent, depending on the age group studied, the similarity in the exposure observed in adults and predicted levels in children, and anticipated impact of treatment on growth and development.

When new pharmacovigilance guidelines (European Medicine Agency, 2012) came into force in EU in July 2012, EMA has issued pharmacovigilance guideline dedicated to paediatric population (European Medicine Agency, 2017b), which provides principal approach on safety collection and assessment in paediatric patients. As compared with clinical trials in the adult population, safety monitoring is expected to be more intensive and thorough in paediatric clinical studies, regarding the number of safety parameters to be collected and the frequency of the measurement/collection points, due to different susceptibility of children to adverse reactions.

In addition, objective and standardised measurement tools, such as scores and scales, should be utilised in the paediatric population, to facilitate safety assessment and reporting.

Adverse event reporting may vary significantly between the age groups. While teenagers and adolescents are expected to cooperate and adequately report all complains they may experience in relation to treatment, in younger children, safety reporting should rely on more wide-ranging methods, such as parental observations and remarks, physical examination, dedicated scores and scales, laboratory tests, vital signs, ECG records, imaging procedures, and other diagnostic methods.

Assessment performed at baseline usually includes general demographic data, physical and mental examination, information related to the primary disease, laboratory tests, vital signs, and ECG. Apart from that, the overall development status, including sexual maturity, should be considered in all paediatric clinical studies. Tanner staging is a commonly used tool for this purpose, which provides information on the progress of puberty (Marshall and Tanner, 1969, 1970).

Clinical chemistry and haematology panels used in paediatric population should include parameters not only relevant to the disease area and drug tested but also suitable for the age group and gender. Adequate reference ranges for all laboratory parameters tested should be applied for the age group(s) involved in the study. Same principals should be considered for all other safety parameters, such as vital signs, body weight, BMI, ECG, and EEG. It is well known that normal ranges for blood pressure and pulse rate, for instance, are different across paediatric age groups and tend to 'evolve' as the child develops.

12.4 ADRs in paediatric population

Internationally agreed definition of adverse events, serious adverse events, and adverse drug reaction are applicable to both adult and paediatric population (European Medicine Agency, 2017a).

In general, paediatric population is more susceptible to ADRs compared with adults. ADRs in paediatric population need specific evaluation, as they may differ in type, frequency, severity, and seriousness from the adult population. Even looking only at paediatric population, there is an intrinsic variation that exists across age groups. What is safe for adolescents may be less safe or even harmful to infants.

- ADRs in paediatric population are different compared with adults, in terms of type, frequency, severity, and seriousness.
- Maturational status has an impact on the response to the medication, in terms of both efficacy and safety
- Medicines can have potential harmful long-term effect on developing organs and potential for causing ADRs with a long latency.
- Risk of medication error is higher in children

Many factors have an impact on the occurrence of adverse reactions in the paediatric population (European Medicine Agency and Committee for Medicinal Products for

Human Use, 2007). Maturational status of organ systems during development stages appears to be of highest importance, as it can directly influence and alter pharmacokinetics and pharmacodynamics of the drug used. This is reflected in the liver and renal system maturation and blood–brain barrier for centrally acting drugs. Further, growth and changes in body mass can have an impact on drug distribution and susceptibility to dose-related adverse reactions. The overall long-term effect of the drugs on developing organs and potential for causing adverse reactions with long latency is difficult to estimate. Finally, not only active substance can be associated with adverse events, but also potentially other excipients may cause harmful effects to the immature organs.

ADRs occur not only during regular labelled use of the drug but also due to errors in medication administration. Paediatric population is associated with higher risk of medication error compared with adults, due to several reasons. One of the key causes of medication error in children is a wrong dose calculation, which is based on body weight or surface, which is, in particular, relevant for drugs with narrow therapeutic window, where a tiny fraction of adult dose is sufficient for children (Ghaleb and Barber, 2010). Inappropriate medicine formulations for paediatric use, which required adjustments, such as dissolving the tablets or dilutions of adult strengths, are another common cause of medication error in children.

12.5 Safety monitoring in paediatric psychopharmacological clinical trials

As seen for recently made available treatments in various therapeutic areas, the use of psychopharmacological treatments in children has substantially increased over the past decade. Due to a need for better understanding of the effect size and potentially harmful effects of drugs in children suffering mental diseases, the number of paediatric clinical trials with antidepressants, antipsychotics, and psychostimulants has increased over the past 10 years (Corell and Kratochvil, 2011).

In clinical studies within psychopharmacology, scoring systems and scales are broadly used to objectively assess specific aspects of the course of the disease and effect of drugs. These instruments are commonly available for adult patients, but only to a certain extent adjusted and validated for paediatric population. Like for the efficacy assessments, an effort should be made to assess the safety profile of investigational products objectively. Careful selection of the safety scales and age-appropriate questioners should be made for children. In case there is no such one available for the age group in a matter, modifications of the adult version can be considered, with the caveat that the scale has not been validated.

One of the commonly used scales assessing safety in paediatric patients treated with psychotropic medication is PAERS. PAERS is a 45- to 48-item questionnaire designed to evaluate any type of adverse event occurring in paediatric patients who are treated with psychotropic medication, primarily as a participant in clinical trials, and was developed as part of the Child and Adolescent Psychiatry Trials Network (CAPTN) (March et al., 2007; Shapiro et al., 2009). PAERS is adverse event elicitation scale used to prospectively collect and investigate adverse events in paediatric clinical trials within psychopharmacology and includes frequency, severity, and causality assessment (Correll and Penzner, 2006). The scale provides useful information on the ADRs typically seen with psychiatric medication, but information on atypical, rare, and serious ADRs is provided to the limited extent. The scale, therefore, complements other more traditional safety assessments, such as self-reported adverse events or other safety scales. All safety methods utilised in one clinical study should be evaluated and presented accurately and transparently, reflecting on the methodology used so that the results can be interpreted in the right context.

Adverse events known as class effects for antidepressants (ADTs) or antipsychotics (APs) that are well described for the adult population can also be seen in children. The paediatric population can be more susceptible to some class effects; hence, adverse event profile of ADTs and APs may differ from the one seen in adults, concerning frequency and severity. The list of most relevant adverse events caused by the second generation of APs includes, but is not limited to, weight gain, metabolic disturbances, neuromotor effects (such as akathisia, restlessness, dyskinesia, and tremor), neuroleptic malignant syndrome (NMS), QT prolongation, hyperprolactinaemia and prolactin-related side effects, sexual dysfunction, and seizures (Henry and Kisicki, 2012).

Differences in pharmacokinetics between children and adults may explain the higher rate of nausea and activation seen with ADTs. Further, some emotional and behavioural side effects of ADTs, such as agitation, hostility, hypomania, and suicidal ideation, have been described.

Risk of suicidal behaviour and treatment with ADTs has been subject to discussion for many years. The US Food and Drug Administration (FDA) has issued warnings that the use of antidepressant medications poses a small but significantly increased risk of suicidal ideation/suicide attempt for children and adolescents. Whether this risk is associated to treatment with ADTs or it is more likely part of the underlying depression or a direct consequence of poorly controlled disease, special attention must be paid to a proper assessment of the risk in clinical trials. The FDA implied a prospective assessment of suicidal behaviour and ideation in 2012 (Department of Health and Human Services and Food and Drug Administration, 2012), and it applies to all clinical trials investigating centrally acting drugs.

Although tremendous progress in paediatric psychopharmacological researches has been observed over the last 10 years, more studies utilising novel principals and technologies are required to better assess safety aspects related to commonly used medications in children suffering mental disorders.

12.6 Challenges and limitations of safety assessment in paediatric clinical studies

There are numerous challenges and obstacles related to the safety evaluation of the drug intended to be used in the paediatric population.

Paediatric clinical studies usually enrol a limited number of patients due to the vulnerability of the population, ethical considerations, or low incidence of the specific condition in children. This consequently results in the small number of patients usually involved in phase I and II clinical studies and even phase III clinical studies in children. Small sample size precludes comprehensive safety evaluation in general and limits to observe anything less than common. Every effort should be therefore made to address these limitations and collect sufficient safety data accurately.

Another obstacle concerns difficulties in study design. Paediatric clinical studies of newer products are usually planned to start very early when data generated in the adult population are not readily available. This consequently creates difficulties in predicting dose or concentration response in the paediatric population, concerning both efficacy and safety.

Apart from adverse event reporting, there are other safety parameters equally important to be investigated, such as laboratory parameters, vital signs, and ECG. Standard laboratory panel is commonly utilised in both adult and paediatric studies. However, since there is a limit on the volume of blood that can be collected, which depends on the age, this may be particularly challenging in paediatric studies involving small children. Besides standard safety and haematology laboratory tests, blood sampling for drug quantification, gene expression profiling, pharmacogenetics, and various biomarkers may be required.

The time required to conduct and complete clinical study in paediatric patients may be substantially longer compared with studies in the adult population. Low recruitment rate and large dropout make it additionally complex and time-consuming. Short-term safety is usually investigated and confirmed in clinical development programme, while long-term effects remain unknown. Postapproval safety studies, that investigate long-term safety in paediatric population, are therefore often implied as postapproval commitment in order to address possible effects on development, such as skeletal, sexual, immune, and psychomotor maturation. Apart from postapproval safety studies, safety data captured in various treatment registries should be considered.

European pharmacovigilance set of guidelines currently in force, also called Good Pharmacovigilance Practice, implies a new conceptual pharmacovigilance process, including risk-management strategies, to be applied early in the life cycle of the product. A risk-management plan is required as a part of marketing authorisation application. This document addresses and summarises all the safety concerns emerged in preclinical and clinical programme of the drug and proposes risk minimisation measure. One domain that is covered by the RMP is a risk in special populations, such as paediatric population. An establishment of the risk-management system early on, which clearly outlines the strategy on safety and risk assessment already in early phase studies, will provide a solid ground for proactive and systematic evaluation of the benefit–risk in all target populations where the product is expected to be used.

- Rare ADRs difficult to detect in small samples
- Long-term safety insufficiently assessed in preapproval phase; postapproval safety studies usually required
- Blood sampling and blood volume collected in minors should be carefully considered

12.7 Safety oversight, independent monitoring

Involvement of external independent groups with appropriate expertise in clinical development programmes, usually called data monitoring committee (DMC) or data and safety monitoring board (DSMB), provides an additional element to the safety monitoring of the trial participants. Independent oversight of clinical trials, monitoring of safety, and integrity of data is warranted in all circumstances where trials involve fragile population, such as paediatric population.

DMC provides advice related to the safety of the subjects enrolled and those yet to be recruited to the trial, as well as the continuing validity and scientific merit of the trial (Department of Health and Human Services and Food and Drug Administration, 2006; European Medicine Agency and Committee for Medicinal Products for Human Use, 2005). DMC performs the review of cumulative safety data, on a regular basis throughout clinical trial(s) and through interim analysis. If a DMC identifies serious safety findings based on the assessments of data generated in a trial, it can recommend modification, such as a change in dose or dose regimen, or early termination of a trial.

While thorough and adequate safety monitoring is required in all paediatric clinical trials, there is no formal requirement on the establishment of DMC in all trials, according to US regulations, unless the trial is conducted in emergency settings (Code of Federal Regulations (CFR), 2011). A need for DMC should be carefully considered on a case-by-case basis. It is sponsor's responsibility to consider and decide if there is a need for external safety monitoring. Early phase studies conducted in unblinded fashion in a limited number of participants may not require the involvement of a DMC.

12.8 Conclusion

This chapter provides overall aspect on safety management in children, with focus on safety monitoring, safety data collection, and assessment in paediatric clinical studies. Further, more specific reflection on safety in paediatric psychopharmacology research was included. Numerous and different aspects should be considered when planning paediatric clinical trials, such as vulnerability of population, age specificity, maturational stage, and long-term and developmental effects of medicine. Even though enhanced safety monitoring is utilised in clinical studies in children, it is difficult to detect and assess anything other than common drug-related adverse events. Comprehensive safety tools for data collection, such as scales and questioners, have been made available to assist safety evaluation. All this has improved safety assessment of medications for use in children, but more research and advanced methodology seems still required in this field.

References

Code of Federal Regulations (CFR), 50.24(a)(7)(iv), 2011. https://www.accessdata.fda.gov/scripts/cdrh/cfdocs/cfcfr/CFRSearch.cfm?fr=50.24.

Corell, C.U., Kratochvil, C.J., 2011. Developments in pediatric psychopharmacology: focus on stimulants, antidepressants, and antipsychotics. J. Clin. Pstchiatry 72 (5), 655–670.

Correll, C.U., Penzner, J.B., 2006. Recognizing and monitoring adverse events of second-generation antipsychotics in children and adolescents. Child Adolesc. Psychiatr. Clin. N. Am. 15, 177–206.

Department of Health and Human Services, Food and Drug Administration, 2006. Guidance for Clinical Trials Sponsors. Establishment and Operation of Clinical Trial Data Monitoring Committee. March.

Department of Health and Human Services, Food and Drug Administration, 2012. Guidance for Industry: Suicidal Ideation and Behavior: Prospective Assessment of Occurrence in Clinical Trials. August.

European Medicine Agency, 2017a. Guideline on Good Pharmacovigilance Practices. Annex I-Definitions. EMA/876333/2011 Rev 4, http://www.ema.europa.eu/docs/en_GB/document_library/Scientific_guideline/2013/05/WC500143294.pdf.

European Medicine Agency, 2012. Good Pharmacovigilance Practice. http://www.ema.europa.eu/ema/index.jsp?curl=pages/regulation/document_listing/document_listing_000345.jsp.

European Medicine Agency, 2017b. Guideline on Good Pharmacovigilance Practices (GVP), Product- or Population-specific Considerations IV: Paediatric Population. http://www.ema.europa.eu/docs/en_GB/document_library/Scientific_guideline/2017/08/WC500232769.pdf.

European Medicine Agency, Committee for Medicinal Products for Human Use, 2005. Guideline on Data Monitoring Committee. July. (EMEA/CHMP/EWP/5872/03 Corr), http://www.ema.europa.eu/docs/en_GB/document_library/Scientific_guideline/2009/09/WC500003635.pdf.

European Medicine Agency, Committee for Medicinal Products for Human Use, 2007. Guideline on Conduct of Pharmacovigilance for Medicines Used by the Paediatric Population. EMEA. CHMP/235910/2005-rev 1, http://www.ema.europa.eu/docs/en_GB/document_library/Scientific_guideline/2009/09/WC500003764.pdf.

Ghaleb, M.A., Barber, N., 2010. The incidence and nature of prescribing and medication administration errors in paediatric inpatients. Arch. Dis. Child. 95 (2), 113–118.

Henry, A., Kisicki, M.D., 2012. Efficacy and safety of antidepressant drug treatment in children and adolescents. Mol. Psychiatry 17, 1186–1193.

March, J., Karayal, O., Chrisman, A., 2007. CAPTN: The pediatric adverse event rating scale. In: The Scientific Proceedings of the 2007 Annual Meeting of the American Academy of Child and Adolescent Psychiatr: 23–28 October 2007; Boston. Edited by: Novins DK, DeYoung, p. 241.

Marshall, W.A., Tanner, J.M., 1969. Variations in Pattern of Pubertal Changes in Girls. Arch. Dis. Child. 44 (235), 291–303.

Marshall, W.A., Tanner, J.M., 1970. Variations in Pattern of Pubertal Changes in Boys. Arch. Dis. Child. 45 (239), 13–23.

Shapiro, M., Silva, S.G., Compton, S., 2009. The child and adolescents psychiatry trials network (CAPTN): infrastructure, development and lessons learned. Child Adolesc. Psychiatry Ment. Health 3, 12.

Sheth, N., 2009. Essentials for starting a pediatric clinical stud (4): clinical pediatric safety planning based on preclinical toxicity studies and pediatric pharmacovigilance guidance. J. Toxicol. Sci. 34, Special Issue II, SP327–SP329.

WHO, 2007. Promoting Safety of Medicine for Children. ISBN 978-92-4-156343-7.

Why do we need to publish paediatric data?

Philippe Auby
Otsuka Pharmaceutical Development & Commercialisation Europe, Frankfurt am Main, Germany

13.1 Introduction

Why should researchers publish their work?

Failure to report and the consequences of not sharing what could be considered as 'vital' information have always been a concern that brought suspicious 'dark clouds' over research.

Historically, specific paediatric use information for medicines utilised in children and adolescents has been lacking. Timely availability of paediatric data also remains a concern.

The 2006 EU paediatric regulation reinforced this need of transparency urging to make paediatric information available to the public and professionals.

13.2 Publishing paediatric data

Please allow us making a "blunt" statement: there are no specificities that would reindeer the process of publishing paediatric data unique.

There could be challenges, like, for instance, finding a journal willing to publish paediatric data that would not necessarily be deemed as the most attractive for their readers. And indeed, there was no open access journal dedicated to child and adolescent mental health until recently. The Child and Adolescent Psychiatry and Mental Health Journal, the first open access electronic journal in this field, was only created in 2007 by Fegert and Vitiello (2007) and became the official journal of the International Association for Child and Adolescent Psychiatry and Allied Professions (IACAPAP, http://iacapap.org/publications).

Additionally, it is important to recognise that nonpublishing negative studies or delaying their publication may result in avoidable risks for patients.

There are fortunately numerous opportunities, not only to be transparent and ethical but also to share lessons learned and data, bringing valuable prescribing information to the field and the public, stimulating exchanges between researchers, and fostering future researches.

13.3 The European paediatric regulation emphasises the need to make paediatric information available to the public

Both Articles 45 and 46 address this need and make publication of the results of the different paediatric studies mandatory for marketing-authorisation holders as one objective of the European regulation is to improve the availability of information on paediatric medicines (https://www.ema.europa.eu/en/human-regulatory/post-authorisation/paediatric-medicines/submitting-results-paediatric-studies).

Article 45 was focusing on all paediatric studies completed by 26 January 2007, that is, the date of entry into force of the Paediatric Regulation, regardless of the study sponsor. For the EMA, "Healthcare professionals and investigators need to be aware of studies that were conducted in the past to avoid unnecessary duplication of trials in children and to raise awareness on efficacy and safety information coming from the past."

Article 46 focuses on paediatric studies that have been completed since the Paediatric Regulation came into force. It requires marketing-authorisation holders to submit information on their sponsored studies within 6 months of completion of each study.

These new requirements of prompt and thorough submission of paediatric study results illustrate well the importance of making paediatric information available sooner than later.

The 10-year EMA general report on the experience acquired as a result of the application of the EU paediatric regulation provides data on new information generated by Article 45 (https://ec.europa.eu/health/sites/health/files/files/paediatrics/docs/paediatrics_10_years_ema_technical_report.pdf).

The table in the succeeding text summarises the recommended SmPC changes related to Article 45 submissions (2008–15) for both centralised and noncentralised approved drugs:

	Article 45 Centralised (EMA-CHMP)	Article 45 Noncentralised (CMDh)
Active substances	62	219
Study reports	199	~19,000
Recommendations for SmPC changes[a] (e.g. addition of paediatric study information or safety data and clarification of paediatric information)	10	~124
New paediatric indications	2	14

[a] Can be more than one change per SmPC.
Source: Procedural and work-sharing documentation of the CMDh, http://www.hma.eu/cmdh.html, using tracking sheet for 31 December 2015. The Co-ordination Group for Mutual Recognition and Decentralised Procedures, Human (CMDh) is a medicine regulatory body representing the EU Member States, Iceland, Liechtenstein, and Norway.

Interestingly during the same period, the share of paediatric trials among all clinical trials increased 2.5-fold, and over 100 PIPs were completed which will consequently generate more information.

Our purpose is not to assess the anticipated outcome of Article 45 in light of the table provided by the PDCO, so we will let our readers make their own opinion, but it should be noted that Article 45 triggered a few new paediatric indications and more than 100 SmPcs updates or clarifications.

So why publishing paediatric data?
To be...
- transparent
- responsible
- influential

Publishing the outcome of paediatric research is also becoming a way to fight back fake scientific news.

Sadly the easy access to medical information via the democratisation of the internet has opened a new area where it can be difficult to distinguish real scientific information to unintentional or malicious misinformation. The current impact of public health is difficult to access.

An exciting pilot Polish study about the spread of fake medical news in social media showed that between 2012 and 2017 revealed that 40% of the most frequently shared links contained text that the authors classified as fake news (Waszak et al., 2018). The authors assessed social media's top shared health web links between 2012 and 2017 in Polish, focusing on the following keywords: "cancer, neoplasm, heart attack, stroke, hypertension, diabetes, vaccinations, HIV, and AIDS". They found that the "most fallacious content concerned vaccines, while news about cardiovascular diseases was, in general, well sourced and informative". While the antivaccine movement is as old as the vaccines themselves, it is interesting to note the importance of technologies and media (internet and social media) in its recent rise, despite overwhelming scientific evidence of the benefits of vaccination.

C.T. Quin and A.J. Rush summarised elegantly in 2009 the benefit for researchers to publish their work, that is, they only exist through the publication of their work: "Writing clearly and accurately is critical to the success of your scientific career. If you do not write clearly, your article will not be cited. If you are not cited, you will not get promoted. If you do not get promoted, you will not have a job. Writing clearly to maximize your likelihood of being cited by others is key to your scientific survival. Published research is your only final product" (Quin and Rush, 2009). Their article provides useful insights on how to write and publish personal research, based on a course that they have taught at the University of Texas Southwestern Medical Center at Dallas. Based on the experience and knowledge they share, it is obvious that publishing paediatric data follow the general rules and that we cannot claim paediatric specificities; however, it emphasises the importance of the "paediatric storyline" using the following table they present in their article.

From Quin, C.T., Rush, A.J., 2009. Writing and publishing your research findings. J. Investig. Med. 57(5), 634–639.

Elements	Place in the manuscript
Gaps in knowledge	Introduction
Hypotheses or questions addressed	Introduction, methods
What was done to test the hypotheses or answer the questions	Methods
The answers to the questions	Results
The meaning of the answers	Conclusions

13.4 The recent rise of the antivaccine movement: Is there a link between vaccination and autism?

The antivaccine movement did not start on social media; it started with vaccination itself. However, its recent rise is concomitant to the development of social media and the Internet. Interestingly the actual trigger was a scientific publication in 1998 by the Lancet, one of the most respected medical journal, of a study suggesting a link between autism spectrum disorders and paediatric vaccination with the measles–mumps–rubella (MMR) vaccine.

The position of the World Health Organization is unambiguous:

> The 1998 study which raised concerns about a possible link between measles-mumps-rubella (MMR) vaccine and autism was later found to be seriously flawed and fraudulent. The paper was subsequently retracted by the journal that published it. Unfortunately, its publication set off a panic that led to dropping immunization rates and subsequent outbreaks of these diseases. There is no evidence of a link between MMR vaccine and autism or autistic disorders (https://www.who.int/features/qa/84/en/).

It is difficult to imagine that the title of Wakefield et al. paper triggered by itself much interest: "Ileal-lymphoid-nodular hyperplasia, nonspecific colitis, and pervasive developmental disorder in children". Despite an uncontrolled design involving a minimal number of children (small sample size of 12), the rather somewhat conclusion of the study created a genuine concern and was extensively utilised by the antivaccine movement.

The logic that the MMR vaccine may trigger autism was questioned because an obvious temporal link as both events, by design (MMR vaccine) and nature (autism spectrum disorder), occur in early childhood (Rao and Andrade, 2011).

Unfortunately, because parents were genuinely concerned, in many countries, MMR vaccination rates began to drop (Hussain et al., 2018). Both the fact that 10 of the 12 coauthors of the paper retracted the conclusion stating that no causal link was established and the fact that no other team was able to replicate these results had no impact. More surprisingly the understanding that Wakefield did not report that he has been funded by lawyers who had been engaged by parents in lawsuits against vaccine-producing companies did not raise any concern. Finally the fact that the patients were specifically chosen for the study because their trajectories suited their case creating an apparent falsification was not much questioned. The antivaccine movement continued to grow based on what some scientists dared to call an 'urban legend', still requiring a lot of efforts from the scientific community to refute a wrong assumption and expose a scientific fraud. Unfortunately, this resulted in public health issues and individual catastrophes. This fraud will probably remain as one of the most severe misconduct in medical history.

What we can learn from this complicated and emotional debate is multiple:

- First, research should never be disconnected from ethical values and scientific rigour.
- Second, interest disclosure should always be made when publishing data.
- Third, in science, understanding the levels of evidence ranking should never be forgotten when concluding on the strength of data generated by research studies.
- Finally, on a specific scientific point of view, to conclude on this complex debate regarding the possibility of a link between childhood vaccinations and the development of autism spectrum disorder, further to the earlier WHO statement, we will report the findings of the meta-analysis performed by Taylor et al. in (2014), strongly suggesting that vaccinations are not associated with the development of autism or autism spectrum disorder:

(1) There was no relationship between vaccination and autism (OR: 0.99; 95% CI: 0.92–1.06).
(2) There was no relationship between vaccination and autism spectrum disorder (ASD) (OR: 0.91; 95% CI: 0.68–1.20).
(3) There was no relationship between [autism/ASD] and MMR (OR: 0.84; 95% CI: 0.70–1.01).
(4) There was no relationship between [autism/ASD] and thimerosal (OR: 1.00; 95% CI: 0.77–1.31).
(5) There was no relationship between [autism/ASD] and mercury (Hg) (OR: 1.00; 95% CI: 0.93–1.07).

13.5 Was the overall publication of paediatric MDD studies with selective serotonin reuptake inhibitors optimal?

During the 1980s the arrival of the SSRIs, which resulted in far fewer side effects than tricyclic antidepressants (TCAs) or monoamine oxidase inhibitors, was welcomed as an essential step in the treatment of mood disorders, not only in adults but also in children and adolescents. Simultaneously the literature on the treatment of MDD in children and adolescents significantly grew up. Nowadays, antidepressants, mainly SSRIs, are quite commonly prescribed in children and adolescents, despite that only fluoxetine is authorised in Europe and the United States for the treatment of depression in children and adolescents and escitalopram in the United States solely for adolescents. Fluoxetine is the only agent to have repetitively shown superiority to placebo on primary efficacy measures in both children and adolescents. Escitalopram, citalopram, and sertraline have also shown superiority over placebo on primary efficacy measures in some studies. All the other antidepressants, that is, duloxetine, paroxetine, venlafaxine, desvenlafaxine, mirtazapine, nefazodone, and selegiline, and even earlier tricyclic antidepressants have not demonstrated any superiority over placebo on the primary efficacy measures. Currently, innovative researches are taking place with two new antidepressants developed in the paediatric population, vortioxetine for children and adolescents with MDD and esketamine nasal spray for MDD in adolescents with imminent risk for suicide (MDSI) (Auby, 2018).

We are discussing in this chapter neither the reasons why SSRIs failed to demonstrate efficacy nor the warnings against their use in younger patients due to concerns of increased risk of suicidal ideation and behaviour as these points have been addressed in previous chapters. Despite such unclear evidence of their benefits versus their risks, the 2007 Cochrane review of selective serotonin reuptake inhibitors (SSRIs) by Hetrick et al. reported that SSRIs were commonly and frequently used in paediatric MDD (Hetrick et al., 2007).

The way paediatric studies of SSRIs in MDD have been published raised several crucial questions:

- the scientific accuracy of the paediatric publications,
- the consequences of the delayed publication of clinical study results,
- the influence of the nonpublished data on the overall assessment of the risks versus the benefits of these drugs.

To look first at the importance of the scientific accuracy of any publication, paediatric or not, we will use the example of the study published in 2001, reporting for the first time the efficacy of a SSRI, that is, paroxetine, and a tricyclic antidepressant, that is, imipramine, with placebo in the treatment of major depressive disorders; this study actually raised a lot of questions (Keller et al., 2001). Like for vaccines, but not as prominent, there is some distrust about the use of antidepressants in paediatric population along with the legitimate concern of not overmedicating children. In this case, we will not discuss here the use of an adult scale, the Hamilton Rating Scale for Depression (HAM-D), as primary endpoint for an adolescent study enrolling young patients from 12 to 18 years of age, as the question of age-appropriate endpoints has been discussed in the methodology chapter; however, the use of an adult scale has been criticised, and the use of the HAM-D has vanished nowadays in paediatric MDD studies. What is interesting here in the discussion of the accuracy of the publication is the discussion around the interpretation of the data following the initial publication. We are going to describe some not well-known controversy and, in this respect, use the quotes for the different authors to help our readers make their own opinion and use this experience for their reflection. The study involved 275 adolescents with MDD who after 1–2 weeks screening period were randomised to an 8-week double-blind period either to paroxetine (20–40 mg), imipramine (gradual upward titration to 200–300 mg), or placebo. The authors reported a high placebo rate in this study, and we have discussed such issue in another chapter (Siegfried K, Indiscriminant efficacy results and the placebo issue). "The protocol described two primary outcome measures: (1) response, which was defined as a HAM-D score of ≤8% or a ≥50% reduction in baseline HAM-D score at the end of treatment, and (2) change from baseline in HAM-D total score. Five other depression-related variables were declared a priori: (1) change in the depressed mood item of the HAM-D; (2) change in the depression item of the K-SADS-L; (3) Clinical Global Impression (CGI) improvement scores of 1 (very much improved) or 2 (much improved); (4) change in the nine-item depression subscale of the K-SADS-L; and (5) mean CGI improvement scores". The following efficacy results were reported: "Of the depression-related variables, paroxetine separated statistically from placebo at endpoint among four of the parameters: response (i.e. primary outcome measure), HAM-D depressed mood item, K-SADS-L depressed mood item, and CGI score of 1 (very much improved) or 2 (much improved) and trended toward statistical significance on two measures (K-SADS-L nine-item depression subscore and mean CGI score)" (Table 2). The response to imipramine was not significantly different from that for placebo across any of the seven depression-related variables. "But paroxetine did not separate statistically from placebo for K-SADS-L depression subscore, mean CGI score, or HAM-D total score". The authors concluded that paroxetine was effective for MDD in adolescents.

In a letter to the editor, Jureidini (Jureidini and Tonkin, 2003) questioned the robustness of the efficacy conclusion based on the fact that the definition of response was changed after the perprotocol statistical analysis, therefore enabling post hoc analysis to show treatment effectiveness. In response, as emphasised in Hetrick et al. in the SSRI Cochrane review (Hetrick et al., 2007), Keller changed the claim of finding a significant effect to stating that the findings showed a strong signal for efficacy (Keller, 2003).

Furthermore, in 2015, a new analysis of this paediatric study was published by a group of authors, including J. Jureidini, who commented on the initial publication (LeNoury et al., 2015). This reanalysis was performed under the restoring invisible and abandoned trials (RIAT) initiative (Doshi et al., 2013). The RIAT initiative is based on a couple of concerns, one being that distorted representations that occur when publications in medical journals present a biased or misleading description of the design, conduct, or results of clinical studies influence practices with scientifically invalid conclusions. They did a thorough reanalysis of the raw data, and their conclusions differ from the original paper: "Our RIAT analysis of Study 329 showed that neither paroxetine nor high dose imipramine was effective in the treatment of major depression in adolescents, and there was a clinically significant increase in harms with both drugs. This analysis contrasts with both the published conclusions of Keller and colleagues and the way that the outcomes were reported and interpreted in the CSR. We analysed and reported Study 329 according to the original protocol (with approved amendments)". Actually the key difference between the efficacy outcomes reported by these authors and the initial publication is linked to the fact that the RIAT initiative "kept faith with the protocol's methods and its designation of primary and secondary outcome variables". We refer our readers to all these publications and want to emphasise the need to ensure that the scientific accuracy of the publication (paediatric or not) cannot be questioned.

The consequences of the delayed publication of clinical study results have also been a concern raised by the RIAT initiative, looking at what they called 'invisibility' which is the fact that a study remains unpublished years after completion.

Delayed in publishing can lead to outdated therapeutic recommendations; therefore the RIAT initiative proposed the following for restoring invisible and abandoned trials:

---

1. Obtain clinical study reports and any other study data
2. Collect documentation of trial abandonment
   For unpublished trials—no primary publication detected by systematic search of the literature and/or confirmation from original trial sponsor or current responsible party that no publication exists
   For misreported trials—evidence of misreporting (ideally, published letters or other articles in the scientific literature or documentation of communication with the original trial publication author(s) detailing the misreporting) and a failure to correct the scientific record
3. Issue a "call to action" by publicly registering your possession of data sufficient for publication
   At least initially, this should be by an electronic response to this article and should include, as a minimum, trial identifiers, number of participants, date completed, publication status, pages in your holding, and level of access to trial data. This declaration offers original sponsors and trialists an opportunity to publish or formally correct their studies within the next 365 days. Send a copy of the rapid response by email to trial sponsors (and authors, for published trials), requesting confirmation of receipt
4. Collect documentation of the need for restoration
   Save time-stamped copies of all rapid responses to this article (or other relevant websites) to document the time elapsed and consequent need for third-party restoration
5. Presubmission inquiry to RIAT friendly journal
   Present editors with documentation from steps 1–4 and seek confirmation of editors' interest
6. Prepare and submit manuscript according to RIAT procedures
   - Include explanation (with references) in the introduction of why this trial is being restored
   - Provide auditable record of decisions (use RIATAR template), documenting which parts of the clinical study report (page number and paragraph) were used
   - Report analyses specified in protocol
   - Denote any analyses that were not prespecified
   - Make all underlying data available electronically

Finally the influence of the nonpublished data on the overall assessment of the risks versus the benefits of any drug is also an important aspect to consider. The systematic review of published versus unpublished data of SSRIs in paediatric MDD conducted by Whittington et al. (2004) released in 2004 concluded that published data suggest a favourable risk–benefit profile for some SSRIs while the addition of unpublished data indicates that except for fluoxetine, risks could outweigh benefits of paroxetine, sertraline, and citalopram: "Our analysis of published data from two trials of fluoxetine suggested a favourable risk-benefit profile for the treatment of depression in children and young people; unpublished safety data lent support to this view. Published data from one trial of paroxetine and two trials of sertraline suggested equivocal or weak positive risk-benefit profiles; however, in both cases, the addition of unpublished data indicated that risks outweighed benefits. Further, our analyses of unpublished data from two trials of citalopram and two trials of venlafaxine suggested unfavourable risk-benefit profiles".

This elegant paper emphasises that nonpublication of clinical study data or omission of important data from published studies can lead to inaccurate therapeutic recommendations.

Obviously, scientific publications in peer-reviewed journals influence physicians' clinical and therapeutic decisions directly and indirectly via the development of clinical practice guidelines. Even if some researches show that clinical practice guidelines have a modest influence in changing physicians' practices, guidelines are now considered as one of the foundations of efforts to improve healthcare. Randomised clinical trials play an essential role for guideline developers as being high in the grading of the strength of evidence, and therefore nonpublication of study data can compromise the quality of the guideline recommendations.

13.6 Conclusion

Publishing promptly ethical and scientifically accurate paediatric research data and therefore being transparent, responsible, and influential should be the legacy of all researchers to inform the public and the professionals. Fostering reflexions and exchanges based on solid data, strong hypothesis, and thorough discussions with professionals and patients' associations will continue enabling innovative paediatric research. Fighting 'fake news' and misinterpretations of paediatric research will probably need more considerations as research outcomes are no longer reserved to a few scientists. Ultimately the goals of bringing better medicines, more precise and hopefully individualised therapeutic strategies, and better preventive interventions will improve the lives of children and adolescents worldwide.

References

Auby, P., 2018. Regulatory spotlight session: development of medicines in child and adolescent psychiatry. In: Industry Perspective, ECNP 2018, Barcelona.

Doshi, P., Dickersin, K., Healy, D., Swaroop Vedula, S., Jefferson, T., 2013. Restoring invisible and abandoned trials: a call for people to publish the findings. BMJ 346, f2865. https://doi.org/10.1136/bmj.f2865.

Fegert, J.M., Vitiello, B., 2007. Peer-reviewed, high quality, worldwide information on all topics relevant to child and adolescent mental health. Child Adolesc Psychiatry Ment Health 1, 1. https://capmh.biomedcentral.com.

Hetrick, S.E., Merry, S., McKenzie, J., Sindahl, P., Proctor, M., 2007. Selective serotonin reuptake inhibitors (SSRIs) for depressive disorders in children and adolescents. Cochrane Database of Syst. Rev. (3). Art. No.: CD004851. https://doi.org/10.1002/14651858.CD004851.pub2.

Hussain, A., Ali, S., Ahmed, M., 2018. The anti-vaccination movement: a regression in modern medicine. Cureus 10 (7), e2919. https://doi.org/10.7759/cureus.2919.

Jureidini, J., Tonkin, A., 2003. Comment on efficacy of paroxetine in the treatment of adolescent major depression: a randomized, controlled trial. J. Am. Acad. Child Adolesc. Psychiatry 42 (5). author reply 514-515.

Keller, M.B., 2003. Paroxetine treatment of major depressive disorder. Psychopharmacol. Bull. 37 Suppl 1, 42–52.
Keller, M.B., Ryan, N.D., Strober, M., Klein, R.G., Kutcher, S.P., Birmaher, B., Hagino, O.R., Koplewicz, H., Carlson, G.A., Clarke, G.N., Emslie, G.J., Feinberg, D., Geller, B., Kusumakar, V., Papatheodorou, G., Sack, W.H., Sweeney, M., Wagner, K.D., Weller, E.B., Winters, N.C., Oakes, R., Mccafferty, J.P., 2001. Efficacy of paroxetine in the treatment of adolescent major depression: a randomized, controlled trial. J. Am. Acad. Child Adolesc. Psychiatry. 40 (7), 762–772.
LeNoury, J.L., Nardo, J.M., Healy, D., Jureidini, J., Raven, M., Tufanaru, C., Abi-Jaoude, E., 2015. Restoring Study 329: efficacy and harms of paroxetine and imipramine in treatment of major depression in adolescence. BMJ 351, h4320 https://doi.org/10.1136/bmj.h4320.
Quin, C.T., Rush, A.J., 2009. Writing and publishing your research findings. J Investig Med. 57 (5), 634–639.
Rao, T.S., Andrade, C., 2011. The MMR vaccine and autism: sensation, refutation, retraction, and fraud. Indian J. Psychiatry 53 (2), 95–96.
Taylor, L.E., Swerdfeger, A.L., Eslick, G.D., 2014. Vaccines are not associated with autism: an evidence-based meta-analysis of case-control and cohort studies. 32 (29), 3623–3629.
Waszak, P.M., Kasprzycka-Waszak, W., Kubanek, A., 2018. The spread of medical fake news in social media – the pilot quantitative study. Health Policy Technol. 7 (2), 115–118.
Whittington, C.J., Kendall, T., Fonagy, P., Cottrell, D., Cotgrove, A., Boddington, E., 2004. Selective serotonin reuptake inhibitors in childhood depression: systematic review of published versus unpublished data. Lancet 363, 1341–1345.

Further reading

WHO, https://www.who.int/features/qa/84/en/.

Conclusion

While the lack of available paediatric medicinal products is not the only major important worldwide public health issue, the lack of 'better medicines for children' remains an obstacle to ensuring optimal child health globally.

Despite the inception of modern psychopharmacology being probably of paediatric nature with Charles Bradley's 1937 breakthrough observation, a significant gap between adult and paediatric psychopharmacology does exit along with significant unmet needs for pharmacological treatments and prevention strategies of psychiatric disorders in children and adolescents.

We are fortunate that Chance, a person with autism, has accepted sharing his story both as a 7-year-old child and now as an adult. Further to making our readers 'feeling' the burden of childhood neuropsychiatric and developmental disorders, his contribution is the very reason why we decided to write this book. We need to listen more to the patients' voices.

Paediatric drug development is indeed not just about being compliant with regulatory obligations. It is about making a meaningful change for children worldwide.

Triggered by international paediatric regulations and digital innovations, we believe that more research will take place in the field of child and adolescent psychiatry.

We are not candid; medical research has a horrible dark history as reflected in the ethical concerns that constitute one storyline of this book.

Coming from different backgrounds and experiences but animated by a similar ambition, this book proposes an overview of paediatric development in the field of child and adolescent psychiatry, offering more 'food for thoughts' than 'simple recipes'.

Twelve chapters focus on the historical, ethical, scientific, regulatory, and operational aspects of paediatric development trying to maintain a fair balance between updated information and constructive criticism. The path taken is paediatric psychopharmacology, but the concepts are universal.

I would like to express my heartfelt thanks to all my co-authors for their great support and dedication, Geneviève Michaux, Beatrice Stirner, Anna I. Parachikova, Jelena Ivkovic, Karel Allegaert, Deborah Lee, and Chance, with a particularly emotional thought to my late friend Klaudius Siegfried, whose generosity, energy, and intellectual curiosity were instrumental in making this book a reality.

We modestly hope our contribution will help 'dreaming', thinking, innovating, and acting 'better medicines for children'.

Index

Note: Page numbers followed by *f* indicate figures, *t* indicate tables, and *b* indicate boxes.

A

Academic associations, 176
ADAPT trial, 104–105
Adverse event reporting, 185–186
Advertising for clinical studies, 164–165
Age-appropriate paediatric formulations, 101
Age-related differences in pharmacokinetics and pharmacodynamics, 104
Age-specific stratifications in studies with mixed children/adolescent groups, 166–167
Amendment to SmPC, 50–51
American medical community, 86
American Psychiatric Association, 7, 8*t*
Amphetamine, 68
Antidepressants, 2, 6
Antipsychotics in adolescents and young adults, 7
Antivaccine movement, 194–195
Assay sensitivity, 125
Attention deficit hyperactivity disorder (ADHD), 5–6, 67
　patient management, 67–68
　symptomatology, 67–68
Autism, 178–179

B

Baseline score inflation, 135
Behavioural aspects of attention and impulsivity, 72–73
Behavioural disorders, 7
Belmont Report, 86–88, 87*t*
Best Pharmaceuticals for Children Act (BPCA), 16, 22, 25–26
Bioinformatics, 71
Biomedical and social impact, 2
Biomedical research ethics, 84
Bipolar I disorder, 7
Brief psychosocial treatment, 160

C

Caregiver engagement, 114
Case record forms (CRFs), 169
Child and adolescent psychiatry, 1
Child and adolescent psychopharmacology
　animal models, 71
　challenges in, 70
　ethical barriers, 71
　off-label use, 71
　preclinical data, 71
　prevalence, 67
　secondary prevention, 67
　unmet needs in, 70–71
Child Assent process, 94–95
Children Depression Rating Scale-Revised (CDRS-R), 107
Clinical assessments, 107
Clinical chemistry and haematology panels, 185
Clinical CPT assay, 73–74
Clinical development programmes, 183–184
　safety and tolerability, 184–185
Clinical Global Impression of Improvement (CGI-I), 128–130, 196–197
Clinical protocol design, 113
Clinical research networks, 114
Clinical studies, 3
Clinical trials, 9
　design and practices, 2
Cognitive-behavioural therapy (CBT), 6, 104–105
Committee for Medicinal Products for Human Use (CHMP), 103–104
Common Protocol Template (CPT), 107
Conflict of interest, 96
Continuous performance tasks (CPT), 73
Contraceptive medication for female adolescents, 167–168
Country and site distribution plan, 154
Country and site selection, 160–163

Cross-species translational knowledge, behavioural and neurobiological levels, 71
Cultural differences, 96

D

Data exclusivity
 and marketing protection, 44–45
 orphan medicinal products, 65
Data monitoring committee (DMC), 110, 189
Data safety monitoring board (DSMB), 110
Declaration of Geneva, 84, 85t
Declaration of Helsinki, 117
Delayed discounting task (DDT), 74
Developmental physiology, 114
Developmental psychopharmacology, 70
Digital revolution, 2–3
Digital therapies, 75
Disease severity, 144
Dose-finding and safety studies in paediatric patients, 12

E

Empiric selection strategies, 144
Enrichment strategies for clinical trials, 144
Escitalopram, 6, 130
Ethical sound paediatric recruitment strategy, 113–114
Ethics Committee (EC) submissions and study approvals, 155–156
Ethics, historical perspective, 81–88
European Medicines Agency (EMA), 39, 119
European paediatric regulation, 7, 27–33, 191–194
 indication *vs.* condition, 28–31, 30t
 paediatric use marketing authorisation, 33
 waivers and deferrals, 31–32
European Patent Convention (EPC), 59
European pharmacovigilance set of guidelines, 188
Evidence-based treatment in paediatric psychopharmacology, 123
Extrapolation, children, 9–10

F

False-negative indiscriminative studies, 125, 127–132
FDA (Food and Drug Administration), 174–176
FDA Paediatric Advisory Committee, 34
FDA pediatric study decision tree, 10, 10f
FDA Safety and Innovation Act (FDASIA), 16
Feasibility assessments, 155
 for study planning, 163, 165–166
Financial incentives or rewards, 8
Fluoxetine, 6
Food and Drug Administration Safety and Innovation Act (FDASIA), 22, 25
Frontostriatal networks, 72–73
Functional gene networks, 71

G

Generalised anxiety disorder (GAD), 6
Generalised off-label prescriptions, 5
Genetic and experimental approaches, 71
Global paediatric development strategy, 35–36

H

Hamilton Rating Scale for Depression (HAM-D), 196–197
Healthcare professionals, 115–116
Health-care utilisation assessments, 168
Health technology assessments, 177

I

ICH E11 'Clinical Investigation of Medicinal Products in the Paediatric Population', 18–19, 18–20t, 99–102, 100–101t
ICH-E11 R1, paediatric drug development, 89, 90t
Impulsivity in ADHD, 74
Independent Ethics Committees (IECs), 93–94
Indiscriminative false-negative studies, 125
 clinical efficacy studies, 145–146
 clinical scale and assessments, 142–143
 error variance of efficacy assessments, 145–146
 health improvement expectations development, 143
 increased variability of outcome measures, 142–143
 in paediatric psychopharmacology, 143–146, 146t
 quality of clinician/investigator–patient interactions, 143

Informed consent, 113
Initial paediatric study plans (iPSP), 22
Institutional Review Boards (IRBs), 93–94, 158–160
Integrated paediatric development in EU and US, 34–35
International Children's Advisory Network (iCAN), 117–118
International Society for Pharmacoeconomics and Outcomes Research (ISPOR), 107, 108*t*
Intransigent ethics and science, 3
Issues of convenience and concerns, 117–118

K

Kiddie Schedule for Affective Disorders and Schizophrenia for School-aged Children, Present and Lifetime Version (K-SADS-PL–DSM-5), 106

L

Local regulatory authorities and IRBs/ECs, 158–160

M

Major depressive disorder (MDD), 6
   epidemiological studies, 1–2
   with selective serotonin reuptake inhibitors, 195–199
Mandatory paediatric obligation, 41
Market exclusivity, 43–45
   authorised orphan medicinal product, 55–56
   reduction of, 57
   reward for a patented orphan medicinal product, 56–57
   substantive and procedural requirements, 53
Marketing authorisation applications (MAA) and applications, 39
Marketing protection, 44–45, 51–52
MDD with imminent risk for suicide (MDSI), 104–105, 195–196
Medical research, 81–82
Medication approval, controlled studies, 70
Mental health disorders, 67
   in children and adolescents, 5
Model-informed drug development (MIDD), 11

Model-informed drug discovery and development (MID3), 11–12, 11*f*
   MID3-related/MID3-enabled guidelines, 11*f*, 12
Modelling and simulation (M&S), 9, 11–12
Monoamine oxidase inhibitors, 195–196

N

National Comorbidity Survey-Adolescent Supplement (NCS-A), 1–2
National patent offices (NPO), 40
National Vaccine Injury Compensation Program (VICP), 15–16
Neurobiological findings and models, 136–137
New Drug Applications (NDAs), 22
Next-generation precision-based treatment, 74
Nonclinical assessments, 109
Nuremberg Code, 82–84, 83*t*

O

Objective and standardised measurement tools, 185
Obsessive-compulsive disorders (OCD), 7
Operational impact of study protocol features, 153–156, 165–169
Operational tasks and study management, 156
Optional paediatric obligation, 42
Orphan designation, 51
Orphan medicinal products, data exclusivity, 65
Orphan Regulation, 40

P

Paediatric bipolar I disorder, 7
Paediatric development programmes, 10–11
Paediatric efficacy MDD studies, antidepressants, 103–104
Paediatric investigation plan (PIP), 39
Paediatric Labeling Rule, 16
Paediatric obligation, 39
   application of, 41–42
   exemptions from, 42
   mandatory, 41
   optional, 42
   and procedure, 40
Paediatric phase 2 pharmacokinetic and tolerance study, 130–131

Paediatric regulations, 40, 119
  2006 EU paediatric regulation, 16–17
  history of, 15–21, 18f
  US paediatric regulation, 15–16
Paediatric research, adult development, 6
Paediatric Research Equity Act (PREA), 16, 22–25, 24t
Paediatric rewards, 40, 42–59
  procedural requirements, 46
  requirements, 45–46
  substantive requirements, 45–46
  types, 45
Paediatric supplementary protection certificate (P-SPC), 63–64
Paediatric trials on trial, 118–119
Paediatric use marketing authorisation (PUMA), 33, 39–40, 45
  application, 53–54
Parental informed consent, 94, 116–117
Patient advocacy, 174–176
Patient availability and recruitment, paediatric psychopharmacology trials, 156–158
Patient/caregiver/caregiver perspective, 173–174
  academic associations, 176
  pharmaceutical companies, 176–177
  regulatory agencies, 174–176
Patient recruitment strategies, 156, 163–165
  advertising for clinical studies, 164–165
  co-morbidity, 166
  competitive vs. noncompetitive, 163–164
  rating trends and biases, 170
  with stratified patient subgroups, 164
  and study conduct challenges, 170
  times, 160–163
Patient-reported outcomes (PROs), 107
Payer groups (health technology assessments), 177
PDCO review procedure, 37
Perceived (artificial) placebo effects, 134–135
Pharmaceutical companies, 176–177
Pharmacological treatment for mental illnesses, 70
Placebo-controlled clinical studies, 131–132
  in adult and paediatric populations with mental disorders, 132–134, 133t
  explanatory value of expectancy theory, 137–138
  factors of, 134–143
  health improvement expectations, 140
  investigator/clinician–patient interaction, 143
  neurobiological development, 140–142
  predisposing factors, 138–139
  in psychiatric indications, 124
  response variance, 142
  situational factors, 139–140
  social environment factors, 139
  suggestibility, 139
  true placebo effects, 135–142, 138t, 141t
Placebo effect, 124–132
Planning of regulatory and Institutional Review Board (IRB), 155–156
Pluripotent stem cells, 71
Pragmatic trial design, 118
Precision medicine, 3
Preclinical 5CSRT assay, 73–74
PSP review procedures and timelines, 37
Psychopharmacological therapies, 1
  ambition and passion, 1
  empirical observations, 1
  sound clinical research, 1
  unmet needs in child and adolescent, 2b
Psychostimulants, ADHD, 5–6, 69
Publishing paediatric data, 191
Pure drug studies vs. studies with combined drug and psychosocial treatment, 167

R

Ready-to-use ethical detailed checklist, 90–91, 94t
Real-world evidence (RWE) studies, 2
Recovery and improved functioning, 70
Recruitment and retention strategies, 113
Recruitment plan (patient), 154
Religious beliefs, 179
Rescue therapy, 110
Restoring invisible and abandoned trials (RIAT) initiative, 197–198
Review PIP procedures and timelines, 37
RNA-based approaches, 71

S

Safety management
  adverse drug reactions, 183
  antidepressants, 187
  antipsychotics, 187
  challenges and limitations, 187–188
  children from unknowns and uncertainties, 183–184
  drug in children, 183

labelling information, 183
oversight, independent monitoring, 189
paediatric development programme, 183
PAERS, 186–187
and tolerability, 184
Schizophrenia, 7
trials, 133
Second-generation antipsychotics (SGA), 5, 7
Selective serotonin reuptake inhibitors (SSRIs), 5, 195–199
Semistructured interview with children, 117
Sequential parallel comparison design (SPCD), 104–105
Serotonin–norepinephrine reuptake inhibitor (SNRI), 130–131
Site and country distribution plan, 154
Site and country selection, 155
Slow recruitment, 110
Social media, 193–194
recruitment, 92, 93t
Source data checking, 169
Stakeholder approach, 114
Stakeholders, paediatric recruitment and retention, 115–118
Study conduct issues in multicentre studies, 156
Study design and methodology
antidepressants, 99
formulations, 109
fundamental paediatric principles, 105–106
long-term care, 109–110
study-specific training, 110
timing of, 109
Study management tasks, 153–156
Study monitoring, 169–171
Study protocol requirements on study feasibility, 165–166
Suicidal behaviour and treatment with ADTs, 187
Supplementary protection certificate (SPC), 39, 43
application content, 52–53
compliance with agreed PIP, 48–50
filing, application, 52
issues with, 54–55
multiple SPCs, 55
with negative term, 54–55

paediatric extension, 62–63
paediatric SPC, 63–64
product approval, 46–48
substantive and procedural requirements, 46–53
Swiss data exclusivity for paediatric medicinal products, 64–65
Swiss paediatric extensions system, 62–64
Swiss paediatric regulatory framework, 21
Swiss Patens Act (PatA), 59–60
Swiss Therapeutic Products Act (TPA), 59–60
Switzerland
bilateral sectoral agreements, 59
data exclusivity, paediatric medicinal products, 61–62
orphan medicinal products, 62
paediatric rewards, types, 61–62
patent-related international treaties and conventions, 59
regulatory framework, 60–61
SPC and paediatric extensions, 61
Swiss paediatric extensions system, 62–64

T

Timing of paediatric studies, 89–90, 90t
Translational clinical-preclinical disease, 72–74
Trial design, 118
Tricyclic antidepressants (TCAs), 104, 195–196
Tuskegee syphilis study, 88

U

Unlicensed or off-label administration of drugs, 114
US paediatric regulatory framework, 22–26
US paediatric voucher, 26–27

W

Willowbrook hepatitis paediatric studies, 88
World Health Assembly, 20
World Health Organization (WHO), 20, 20–21t
World Medical Association, 84–85, 85t

Y

Young Mania Rating Scale (Y-MRS), 107

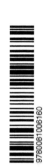